# Cinemeducation

## A comprehensive guide to using film in medical education

Edited by

## Matthew Alexander
*Professor of Family Medicine*
*University of North Carolina School of Medicine*

## Patricia Lenahan
*Associate Clinical Professor*
*Department of Family Medicine*
*University of California*
*Irvine College of Medicine*

## Anna Pavlov
*Assistant Clinical Professor of Family Medicine*
*UCLA School of Medicine*
*Director of Behavioral Science*
*Pomona Valley Hospital Medical Center, California*

Forewords by
Thomas L Campbell
Marian R Stuart

Radcliffe Publishing
Oxford • Seattle

**Radcliffe Publishing Ltd**
18 Marcham Road
Abingdon
Oxon OX14 1AA
United Kingdom

www.radcliffe-oxford.com
Electronic catalogue and worldwide online ordering facility.

---

British Library Cataloguing in Publication Data

A catalogue record for this book is available from the British Library.

ISBN 1 85775 692 4

Typeset by Anne Joshua & Associates, Oxford
Printed and bound by TJ International Ltd, Padstow, Cornwall

# Contents

# Foreword

Recall the scene from *Ferris Bueller's Day Off*, in which his high school economics teacher desperately but futilely tries to engage his disinterested students in the subject. 'Anyone? . . . anyone? . . . anyone?' he inquires, searching for a response whilst his students sleep, shoot spitballs and talk with each other. I have felt like this at times, teaching behavioral science and family systems to a generation of family medicine residents over the past 20 years. Once a week for 50 minutes, I would try to engage a group of 6 to 12 interns and residents, most of whom were sleep deprived (a bit less since the restriction of resident work hours) and distracted by more urgent needs, such as the hospital admissions waiting for their return, the patient treated earlier in the day and labwork to be followed up on. I often consider Maslow's hierarchy of needs when teaching family medicine residents. First, they needed adequate sleep and food. Providing snacks during teaching seminars helps (it's hard to sleep while eating). Next, they need the knowledge and skills to keep their patients alive and do no harm. To be most effective, behavioral science teaching needs to be focused, practical, skills based and, when possible, entertaining. Otherwise one risks facing an unresponsive and half-asleep audience.

I first learned about Matthew Alexander's work using film clips for teaching when I was at the annual STFM Families and Health conference. I had occasionally used film in some of my teaching, but found it difficult to find short segments of a film that illustrated the point that I wanted to make on the topic for the day. Alexander's seminar and work was a gift. He provided specific short film segments for a host of different educational topics, and the counter times to find these segments on video. Anyone who has tried to find such segments knows how laborious this task can be, having to watch the film several times and try to determine when to start and stop each segment.

Alexander's work was first published in *Family Medicine*, where he coined the term 'cinemeducation', and expanded in other papers in *Families, Systems and Health* and *Annals of Behavioral Science and Medical Education*. This edited book is a huge advance and expansion of his previous work and a tremendous resource for medical educators. He is joined, as co-editors, by two other behavioral scientists and experienced medical educators. Over 25 authors from residency programs and medical schools across the country have contributed chapters. There are entire chapters on common behavioral science topics, including normal developmental issues, common psychiatric diagnoses and the physician–patient relationship. Each is packed with examples of film clips that illustrate different aspects of the topic. There are hundreds of film segments listed in this book, with descriptions of each, how they can be used in teaching and, of course, the counter numbers to locate them on video or DVD.

I started using film segments in my teaching on a more regular basis several months after Alexander's first paper on cinemeducation was published. My favorite and most frequently used film for teaching about families and health has been *Dad*, the story of Jake Tremont (Jack Lemmon) and his domineering wife Betty (Olympia Dukakis). Jake has dementia and has become completely dependent upon his wife. Early in the film, she suffers a heart attack, and their adult son Jack (Ted Danson) returns home to help care for his father and assist him in becoming more independent. It is a powerful and humorous film about the impact of an illness on family life and family roles. I have discovered numerous uses for the film, with different audiences ranging from medical educators to medical students and different formats including large lectures and small workshops. I usually ask those in the audience or workshop to imagine that they are this family's primary care physician and consider what they would do to help the family under their current circumstances. We start with a brief family assessment: five components (family structure, development, strengths, problems and health beliefs) in five minutes. Then we can discuss a range of topics that are presented in the film: how to help Betty reduce some of her household tasks (doing laundry, cleaning, etc) after her MI, while still feeling in charge at home; how to help this family cope with the role changes that occur as a result of the illness; how to handle family conflict or a dominating family member during a family interview; what to do when a family member insists that the patient not be told his/her diagnosis.

It is always instructive to talk about what the learners observe from the film and their assessment of the family, but I have found that the most powerful use of film is as a trigger tape for role-plays, as described by Alexander in Chapter 1. This is when the learning really begins. By watching a segment of film, students or residents are able to experience the patient or family and role play the characters more realistically and effectively. The participants experience what it is like to be in a family like the one portrayed. They generally love to play challenging patients or family members, since most of them have cared for such individuals. It is not uncommon for learners to remark 'now I understand why my patients respond this way'. The learner who plays the physician is able to try different approaches with the identified patient and the family in a safe environment where he or she can make mistakes and get feedback from the other participants.

One challenge for the physician interviewing the Tremont family from the movie *Dad* is how to join with Betty, but not let her dominate the interview, so that the physician can learn how Jake is doing and what his concerns and thoughts are. Different learners can try out different approaches in sequence and then get advice from the larger group. One participant may struggle with Betty and attempt to expel her from the exam room to talk with Jake alone. Another may be able to develop a collaborative treatment plan with Betty, something the first learner could not have believed possible. With such role plays, the teacher can control the difficulty of the interview, depending upon the goals of the teaching session and the skills of the learners. With the same scenario, one can instruct those role playing the Tremont family to be compliant and supportive for inexperienced interviewers or become resistant and angry when teaching this approach to medical educators. The participants usually have a great time with this exercise and come away with some new skills and less afraid of interviewing a challenging or conflictual family.

Few learners, even the most resistant resident who doesn't believe in 'all this touchy-feely stuff', can resist the magic of movies. Teaching sessions are often transformed when the lights are dimmed and the characters come alive, even for a short segment of film. Perhaps the most powerful effect of movies is that they engage the learners' feelings, which is critical to effective learning. When one becomes emotionally engaged in a subject or an interaction, the potential for learning is greatly increased. The educational material starts to make a difference, and new information or new skills are more likely to be learned and retained.

Using films clips can be an effective way to include humor in medical teaching. Like other emotions, generating humor or laughter often makes learners more open and receptive to new material. Much of medicine and medical education is serious stuff, often dry and sometimes boring. Those of us who teach the psychosocial aspects of medicine sometimes take ourselves and our topics too seriously, as if we are trying to compete with those teaching biomedicine by proving that our topic is just as serious and thus important. Adding humor to our teaching helps students to become more relaxed, even playful, and willing to attempt new skills and integrate new knowledge. Many film makers have skillfully incorporated humor into films about very painful and sensitive topics, such as death and dying.

Somatizing patients are one of the most challenging types of patients for clinicians. These patients frustrate our attempts to 'fix' their physical complaints. Students and residents universally enjoy the film clip from *Hannah and Her Sisters* in which Mickey (Woody Allen) is evaluated for ringing in his ears and becomes convinced that he has a brain tumor. The clinician can identify with the clumsy attempt by Mickey's physician to reassure him. 'If there is nothing seriously wrong with me, why are you doing all these tests' says Mickey. 'Trust me' replies his physician. If only the hypochondriacal patient could 'trust' his/her physician's reassurance. So instead, students or residents can practice how they would respond to Mickey's insecurity.

With such a powerful teaching tool that taps into the learners' emotional world, there must be some potential risks of using film clips for teaching. The biggest risk occurs when a film clip deals with an unresolved and painful issue of one of the learners. For example, some students or residents have experienced the early and sometimes tragic death of a parent or sibling. A film about such a death can be very difficult for the learner to watch and discuss. I recently saw the movie *Ray*, the biography of Ray Charles, which highlights the lifelong impact on him of the accidental drowning of his younger brother. I warned a friend whose younger sibling had drowned in a similar fashion about the content of the movie. If this friend had seen the movie in an educational setting and been asked to discuss it in a group setting, the experience might have been quite distressing. These are experiences that most behavior science teachers must often address in all their teaching, but the effect may be more powerful because of the emotional impact of film.

I expect that this book will stimulate a significant increase in the use of film clips in medical education, at medical schools, residencies and with continuing professional education. I have already started my lists of films to see, DVDs to buy and film segments to use during future lectures and seminars. I can envision medical educators wandering the aisles of Blockbusters with this book in hand, looking for the film for that week's teaching session. If only Ferris Bueller's unfortunate high school teacher had been able to access this book.

Thomas L Campbell MD
William Rocktaschel Chair and Professor of Family Medicine
Associate Director, URMC Center for Primary Care
University of Rochester School of Medicine and Dentistry
*November 2004*

# Foreword

Today, more than ever before, the fact that social and psychological factors significantly influence the state of patients' health and illness is widely accepted. An emerging body of knowledge exploring the relationship between mind and body supports our understanding that these entities are not operating in isolation but rather are fully integrated and communicate bidirectionally. Whatever impacts one also impacts the other. Medical educators, however, face several obstacles when trying to integrate these concepts into the curriculum in a meaningful way. Students and residents are generally more comfortable focusing on the biomedical aspects of a case. They want to learn about the aspects of disease, of the differential diagnosis and the pharmacological fixes that can be prescribed. Dealing with the emotional factors that a patient may be experiencing can be quite daunting, especially if students are uncomfortable with their own emotional reactions stirred up by the situation.

When learners do not feel safe in the emotional arena, it is hard for them to see the importance of addressing psychosocial issues. In fact, they will often not even recognize the existence of these issues. Sensitizing our learners to the range of emotional reactions to be expected in a variety of human situations becomes a prerequisite for teaching counseling skills. Cinemeducation encourages the development of psychosocial competencies by providing an effective medium for focusing on exactly the situations we wish to explore. Movies are perfect for capturing learners' attention. Learners are able to identify with the characters on the screen and broaden their awareness of both diverse lifestyles and common human reactions. Powerful scenes evoke powerful reactions. Dramatic images and narratives stimulate genuine, unguarded emotional reactions. They can help to make learners aware of personally relevant biopsychosocial issues, allow them to talk about painful issues in a safe arena and improve empathic abilities.

*Cinemeducation: A comprehensive guide to using film in medical education* is a marvelous tool that is entirely user friendly. Alexander, Lenahan and Pavlov have captured an amazing array of significant small scenes from a large variety of films, cameos illustrating crucial moments and interactions. They have not only organized these scenes into topics that focus on individual and family life cycles, specific clinical entities, the doctor/patient relationship and a variety of special populations, but they provide specific discussion questions that can be used to help learners process the experience. The range of films that are included is comprehensive and, with exact counter numbers provided, simplify the task of the medical educator to plan and present meaningful sessions.

As a behavioral scientist and principal author of *The Fifteen Minute Hour* I have spent the last 25 years teaching interviewing and counseling skills to clinicians at various levels of training. I know how hard it sometimes can be to capture learners' attention and to break through the reluctance to deal with uncomfortable situations. Using the material that can be found in this book, we will all have a much easier and more successful time.

Marian R Stuart, PhD
Clinical Professor
UMDNJ-RWJ Medical School, New Jersey
*November 2004*

# Preface

## Overview

Lights, camera, action!!! Or, for the purposes of this book, perhaps we should say 'Lights, camera and *educational* action!' You are about to be exposed to over 400 *scenes* with their exact counter numbers from 125 *movies* that can be used to teach a broad variety of behavioral medicine, primary care and psychiatry related topics. Additional movies without scenes are also referenced at the end of the book. If you are already using movies in your curriculum, we believe that this book will help you to expand your cinemeducational repertoire. If you are not using movies in your curriculum, we are confident that you will be after reading this book. It has been our experience that integrating movies into teaching improves both learner *and* teacher satisfaction.

Cinemeducation refers to the use of movie clips or whole movies to help educate learners about bio-psycho-social-spiritual aspects of healthcare. Numerous articles and books have already been written about cinemeducation, many of which are cited in this work. To our knowledge, however, this book is unique. No other existing work lists so many *specific scenes* with their *counter numbers* and corresponding trigger questions. We believe that *all* healthcare educators, as well as many liberal arts educators, will find this book of great utility in designing and implementing their curriculum.

The book is meant to be immediately applicable to any relevant educational setting. Each chapter begins with an explanation of why a particular topic is important for healthcare learners. After this introduction, specific movies, scenes (with counter numbers) and trigger questions used for stimulating group discussion are listed under multiple subheadings pertinent to the chapter itself. Each movie and scene listed has a description. Since learners often have not seen the entire movie, we have found these descriptions very important in 'setting up' the scene, and we recommend that they be read aloud before the scene is shown. Wherever possible, readings which the authors have found useful when teaching a particular subject are listed in Appendix 1. Learners may benefit from reading these sources, either before or after the teaching session. Formal references are listed at the end of each chapter. Additional movies that deal with the same subject are included in a comprehensive list of movies suitable for cinemeducation which can be found in Appendix 4 at the end of the book.

Topics in this book are specifically relevant to, but not limited to, learners in the following fields: family medicine, psychiatry, pediatrics, obstetrics and gynecology, medical ethics, physical medicine and rehabilitation, internal medicine, oncology, geriatrics, clinical psychology, counseling psychology, child and adolescent psychology, substance abuse counseling, pastoral counseling, social work, family therapy, law, nutrition and pharmacology. Chapters have been authored by family physician, psychiatrist, psychologist, marriage and family therapy and social work educators.

The book is divided into eight parts. In Part I, we explore the historical context of cinemeducation. In the opening chapter, Dr Alexander provides a review of the literature, including a sampling of specific applications of cinemeducation. In Chapter 2, Dr Silenzio and colleagues describe their academic program with medical students using cinema as part of a narrative medicine curriculum. Their chapter helps to put cinemeducation into a larger context.

In Part II, we identify cinematic film clips used to teach issues relevant to the individual and family life cycle. This part contains chapters on child and adolescent development, adult development, family dynamics, sexuality through the life cycle, chronic illness, geriatric medicine and end-of-life issues.

Part III is devoted to adult diagnostic categories. It provides cinemeducational approaches to many of the most common and debilitating clinical problems treated by healthcare professionals, including post-traumatic stress disorder, anxiety, depression and somatization, chemical dependency, family violence, schizophrenia and bipolar disorders, personality and dissociative disorders, and eating disorders.

Part IV provides film clips to help cinemeducators teach healthcare professionals about important aspects of the doctor–patient relationship. It includes chapters on cinemeducational approaches to teaching interviewing skills, the professional and personal self of the physician, identifying and handling the difficult patient, ethics and human values, medical error and motivating patients to adopt healthy lifestyles.

Part V addresses the use of cinemeducation to teach about specific populations, including gay, lesbian, bisexual and transgendered populations, individuals who align themselves with complementary and alternative medicine, culturally diverse populations, and those with physical and mental disabilities.

Part VI consists of a recent quantitative and qualitative study of graduates exposed to cinemeducation in a healthcare setting.

Part VII contains chapters applicable to teaching about leadership, teamwork and organizational dynamics, and a 'how to' chapter specifically designed to help cinemeducators use the available VCR and DVD technology. We strongly recommend that educators who are not familiar with the use of these technologies refer to this chapter before using this book, which utilizes both VCR and DVD time counters. VCR and DVD time counters closely match one another if VCR time counters are set to zero when studio credits are displayed at the outset of the videocassette.

Finally, in Part VIII, the three editors ponder the future of cinemeducation and make specific suggestions for greater collaboration between *all* cinemeducators.

We also include several Appendices. Appendix 1 lists suggested readings for most of the specific topic areas in the book. These are organized by chapter and subheading. For those interested in conducting graduate surveys of their cinemeducation programs, we include Dr Alexander's questionnaire in Appendix 2. Appendix 3 contains suggestions for building your video library. Appendix 4 includes a list of cinemeducation-related websites, as well as an exhaustive list of selected movies appropriate for cinemeducation. Finally, in Appendix 5, the editors choose their top ten cinemeducation movies *of all time*. At the very end of the book, an index of both topics and movies can be found.

## Getting started

Every cinemeducator needs several things in order to function. First, they require access to movies. In Appendix 3 we provide suggestions for building a cinemeducation library. Second, they need access to appropriate equipment on which to first identify scenes and then play them back for learners. It is *essential* in this regard to have either a VCR or a DVD unit that has time-counter capability, preferably accessible by remote control. For instructions on how to use time counters appropriately, please see Chapter 29 to answer any questions that you might have about using current technology for cinemeducation.

## Caveats

Many novice cinemeducators worry about the legality of using movies for teaching. We believe that the use of movies for teaching purposes is protected under the Fair Use Doctrine. This doctrine, as codified in Title 17, Section 107 of the US Copyright Code, allows copywritten material to be used for non-profit educational purposes. For more information about this doctrine, please see http://fairuse.stanford.edu or go to the Legal Information Institute's website at www4.law.cornell.edu/uscode/17/107. However, we do *not* advise that cinemeducators copy films either in their entirety or in sections, as this *may* constitute copyright infringement. If in doubt, we encourage you to check with a local copyright attorney.

Although this is a *comprehensive* guide to cinemeducation, it is by no means *definitive*. New movies are released constantly, many of which have great application to cinemeducation but which, for obvious reasons, could not be included in this book. Also, many excellent older movies exist that may not have been included. We have tried our best to be as inclusive as possible in this regard by creating an extensive list of selected movies in Appendix 4. These are movies that may not appear in the book text. Also, while we have tried our best to comprehensively address all of the major topics currently taught by behavioral medicine educators, we may have omitted one or more. If a topic that you teach is not included in the table of contents, please check Appendix 4 to see if it is listed there along with relevant movies. However, if your favorite movie or topic is not included in the entire book, we apologize in advance. We have tried, as much as possible, to be fully inclusive.

Every clip in this book has been checked and double-checked both for its utility for teaching and for the accuracy of the scene time provided. However, despite our best efforts, it is our experience that time counters vary from one machine to another by as much as three or more minutes. Consequently, we encourage users of this book to allow extra time to locate scenes *before* class! Once you have found and used a scene for teaching, though, it becomes much easier to find and reuse that scene again. Over time, you may also modify any given scene to suit your own tastes, letting it run either for less time or for longer than we have suggested.

And so, finally, we encourage you to please sit back, pass the popcorn and enjoy the show!

Matthew Alexander
Patricia Lenahan
Anna Pavlov
*November 2004*

# About the editors

**Matthew Alexander** PhD, MA is Professor of Family Medicine at the University of North Carolina School of Medicine, the first psychologist to have achieved this distinction. He is Director of Behavioral Medicine in the Department of Family Medicine at Carolinas Medical Center, Charlotte, North Carolina, and has an active clinical psychology practice, specializing in individual and marital therapy. Dr Alexander has had a long interest in medical humanities, and he coined the phrase 'cinemeducation', which is now a Google search-engine word. He is a distinguished public speaker who has spoken in Europe and throughout the USA on the use of cinema as a teaching tool. His articles on cinemeducation have been published in such professional journals as *Family Medicine, Families, Systems and Health* and the *Annals of Behavioral Science and Medical Education*. Dr Alexander resides in Charlotte, North Carolina, with his wife, Elaine, and their two children, Ethan and Natalie. More information about him can be found at www.alexandertherapy.com

Matthew Alexander
Professor of Family Medicine
Department of Family Medicine
Carolinas Medical Center
Charlotte, North Carolina
Email: matthew.alexander@carolinashealthcare.org

**Patricia Lenahan** LCSW, LMFT received her AM degree from the University of Chicago School of Social Service Administration, and is a licensed clinical social worker and licensed marriage and family therapist. Ms Lenahan is an Associate Clinical Professor at the University of California Irvine College of Medicine and Director of Behavioral Medicine for the Department of Family Medicine. She coordinates the medical school's curriculum in family violence, sexuality and diversity. In addition, she teaches gerontology classes in the extended education program at California State University, Fullerton and serves as faculty for the American Society on Aging's substance abuse and aging program. She is a state-certified domestic violence advocate and a member of the Family Violence Emergency Response Team of the Santa Ana Police Department. Ms Lenahan has published in the areas of family violence, sexuality and diversity, and has lectured on these topics at national and international meetings in Europe, Asia and Africa. She enjoys international travel, reading and film, and is an avid horsewoman.

Patricia M Lenahan
Associate Clinical Professor
Director of Behavioral Medicine
Department of Family Medicine
University of California
Orange, California
Email: pmlenaha@uci.edu

**Anna Pavlov** PhD is a licensed clinical psychologist who has worked in medical education since 1992 when she was a post-doctoral fellow in Primary Care Health Psychology at the Michigan State University College of Human Medicine, Flint Campus. She has been the Director of Behavioral Science at Pomona Valley Hospital Medical Center's Family Medicine Residency Program since 1998, and has an appointment with the UCLA Department of Family Medicine. Dr Pavlov has presented at numerous family medicine forums and has special interests in physician well-being and psychooncology. She lives in Upland, California, with her husband, Jeff Winokur, and enjoys travel, film and theatre.

Anna Pavlov
Assistant Clinical Professor of Family Medicine
UCLA School of Medicine
Director of Behavioral Science
Pomona Valley Hospital Medical Center, California
Email: anna.pavlov@pvhmc.org

# List of contributors

Terry A Allbright MEd, LPC, RNC, LCCE
Faculty Associate
Department of Internal Medicine
Texas Tech University Health Sciences Center
Odessa, Texas
Email: Terry.Allbright@ttuhsc.edu

Pablo Gonzalez Blasco MD, PhD
Scientific Director
SOBRAMFA-Brazilian Society of Family Medicine
São Paulo, Brazil
Email: pgblasco@uol.com.br

Bertie E Bregman MD
Assistant Clinical Professor of Medicine
Columbia University, Center for Family Medicine
New York, New York
Email: bmb26@columbia.edu

James K Burks MD
Professor of Medicine
Programme Director, Internal Medicine
Texas Tech University Health Sciences Center
Odessa, Texas
Email: james.burks@ttuhsc.edu

Kathleen A Culhane-Pera MD, MA
Assistant Professor
Department of Family Practice and Community Health
University of Minnesota
St Paul, Minnesota
Email: kathiecp@yahoo.com

Alexandra Duke DO
Associate Clinical Professor
Department of Family Medicine
UCI Medical Center
Orange, California
Email: aduke@uci.edu

William Elder Jr PhD
Associate Professor of Family Practice
University of Kentucky Chandler Medical Center
Lexington, Kentucky
Email: welder@email.uky.edu

Amy Ellwood MSW, LCSW
Professor, Director of Behavioral Science
University of Nevada School of Medicine
Department of Family Medicine
Las Vegas, Nevada
Email: ellwood@med.unr.edu

Colleen Fogarty MD
Assistant Professor
Department of Family Medicine
University of Rochester
Rochester, New York
Email: colleen_fogarty@urmc.rochester.edu

Kathryn Fraser PhD
Behavioral Science Director
Halifax Medical Center
Family Practice Residency Program
Daytona Beach, Florida
Email: Kathryn.fraser@hmc.halifax.org

Ruth Hart MD
Clinical Associate Professor
Department of Family Medicine
SUNY Upstate Medical University
Syracuse, New York
Email: ruth.h.hart@worldnet.att.net

Sam P Hooper Jr PhD
Assistant Professor
Department of Family and Community Medicine
Texas Tech University Health Sciences Center
Odessa, Texas
Email: sam.hooper@ttuhsc.edu

Craig A Irvine PhD
Administrator, Research and Predoctoral Education Programs
Columbia University, Center for Family Medicine
New York, New York
Email: ci44@columbia.edu

Joe Kertesz MA, LPC
Associate Professor
Department of Behavioral Medicine
University of North Carolina
Wilmington, North Carolina
Email: joe.kertesz@nhhn.org

Heather A Kirkpatrick PhD
Director of Behavioral Science for Internal Medicine
Genesys Regional Medical Center
Grand Blanc, Michigan
Email: koshka@yahoo.com

Wadi Najm MD
Clinical Professor
Department of Family Medicine
University of California-Irvine
Orange, California
Email: winajm@uci.edu

Layne Prest PhD, LMFT
Associate Professor/Director of Behavioral Medicine
Department of Family Medicine
University of Nebraska Medical Center
Omaha, Nebraska
Email: laprest@unmc.edu

Jeffrey Ring PhD
Director of Behavioral Sciences
White Memorial Medical Center
Los Angeles, California
Email: ring@usc.edu

Robert E Sember PhD
Staff Associate
Department of Sociomedical Sciences
Columbia University
New York, New York
Email: res47@Columbia.edu

Vincent MB Silenzio MD, MPH
Assistant Professor of Family Medicine and Community Preventive Medicine
University of Rochester
Assistant Professor of Clinical Sociomedical Sciences
Columbia University
Rochester, New York
Email: w.m.silenzio@rochester.edu

Joan Simpson PsyD
Daymark Recovery Services
Kannapolis, North Carolina
Email: jsimpson@claymarkrecovery.org

Robert Tran MD, MPH
Assistant Clinical Professor
Department of Family Medicine
University of California-Irvine
Orange, California
Email: tranr@uci.edu

Christine Wan MD
Wendover Family Medicine
Odessa, Texas
Email: drawn@cableone.net

Dael Waxman MD
Medical Director, Behavioral Medicine
Department of Family Medicine
Carolinas Medical Center
Charlotte, North Carolina
Email: dael.waxman@carolinashealthcare.org

Jay C Williams PhD, MSW
Clinical Associate Professor
School of Social Work and Department of Psychiatry
University of North Carolina-Chapel Hill
Chapel Hill, North Carolina
Email: jaycwilliams@bellsouth.net

Anthony Zamudio PhD
Director of Behavioral Sciences
California Hospital Medical Center
Los Angeles, California
Email: azamudio@usc.edu

Please note that, although this book is written by American authors, it is published by an English company. Therefore, please be aware that there may be deviations from the usual grammatical style used in America.

# Part I

## Historical context

# Chapter 1

# A review of the literature

*Matthew Alexander*

## Overview

The very first 'moving' picture was used to objectively capture the trot of a horse. One of the interesting ironies of the twentieth century is that rather than becoming the instrument of science for which they were originally intended, 'moving' pictures instead became a vastly popular outlet for our collective imaginations.[1]

Movies allow us to briefly inhabit a conscious dream state, one that is populated by larger-than-life figures engaged in human comedy and drama. While films allow us to *escape* our own worlds for a short period of time, they can *also* provide viewers with profound insights. As Glen Gabbard MD, noted psychiatrist and author of several books on psychiatry and the cinema, has stated, 'Contemporary citizens of the United States learn what it means to be human from the movies.'[2] In a recent essay, noted director Martin Scorsese echoes this theme when he speaks about the universal appeal of cinema's leading men: 'These characters play out feelings we can all relate to. There's an empathy. A character makes a choice, and you think, "I wonder if I would have done it like that?" Maybe in watching them we can find a way out of our private jails, our torment.'[3]

In the past 20 years, healthcare educators have increasingly used popular movies as a curricular tool for teaching psychosocial issues to a wide range of learners, including medical students,[4] counselors,[5,6] nurses,[7] family doctors,[8,9] psychiatrists[10–12] and dentists.[13] Specific content areas addressed by this innovative format include psychology and the law,[14] family systems theory and practice,[15,16] multicultural competency,[17,18] child development,[7] marital, family and group counseling,[5,19] psychiatric diagnoses[20–23] and clinical pharmacology.[24] As further evidence of their broad use in educational and psychological contexts, films are also being used as a tool designed to increase self-awareness and dialogue in various types of psychotherapy.[25,26] One excellent resource, for example, utilizes clips from the movie *The Horse Whisperer* to facilitate therapeutic dialogue between parents and traumatized children.[27]

It is no wonder that films are so adaptable to the educational (and therapeutic) context. First and foremost, movies are fun, entertaining and readily enjoyed by learners. Using the considerable talents of actors, directors, cinematographers and screenwriters, movies offer visual portrayals of life that are memorable and provocative. As such, they easily trigger discussion and provide a useful counter-weight to more traditional didactic ways of teaching. Since individuals portrayed in movies are not 'real' (with the exception of documentaries), healthcare learners can be more honest about their reactions to these characters than they probably would be if they were discussing actual patients. This is an example of 'displacement,' a technique that allows one 'to become emotionally involved in a situation but also . . . to maintain enough distance to maintain objectivity.'[5]

Movies can also expose learners to under-represented patient populations, and may be viewed repeatedly to underscore teaching points. The use of *movie clips in particular* is a very time-efficient teaching tool, since a short film segment can generate hours of discussion. A more in-depth discussion of rationales for the use of cinemeducation can be found in the excellent, but unfortunately out-of-print, book entitled *Movies and Mental Illness: using films to understand psychopathology.*[22]

## Educational approaches using films

A variety of teaching strategies are possible using films and film clips. Perhaps the most common of these strategies is the use of an entire film or film clip(s) to stimulate small group discussion.[4,5,8,9,13,15,17,18] In this approach, the movie or movie clip is shown to the entire group, before or after which educators pose trigger questions tailored to their teaching goals. Teaching points may include general emotional reactions of the viewer, diagnostic impressions, therapeutic and treatment considerations, and associations with one's own professional and personal life.

Zazulak has provided a very useful protocol for educators using cinemeducation.[28] After the viewing of a specific clip, he suggests that a series of questions be asked to allow students to explore their responses in a stepwise fashion, moving from the impersonal to the personal. His protocol includes such questions as the following.

1  What did you see?
2  What did you hear?
3  What did you feel?
4  What did you think?
5  What impact might viewing this clip have on your future clinical encounters?

One particularly innovative use of film to trigger group discussion involves having participants viewing the film clip twice, first with *no sound* and then *with sound*. The resulting discussion is geared toward deepening students' awareness of nonverbal communication and congruence between verbal and nonverbal information, which are important skills for healthcare professionals.[5]

Additional teaching strategies that lend themselves to the use of film include the following:

1  *Role play*. In one educational setting, a clip from the movie *Steel Magnolias* is used to 'set the stage' for a role play. The movie clip in question illustrates family conflict around the issue of diabetic control. After viewing the clip, learners are asked to play the multiple family members portrayed in the film as they engage in a fictional 'family conference' with a physician. This role play allows learners to practice skills that are useful when conducting family conferences, as well as to experience the situation from many different family members' perspectives, a critical skill in effective family counseling.[15]

In another setting, educators construct a history and a mental status examination derived from a selected film character.[22] Learners are then asked to play the part of an expert psychiatric witness in a mock court and base their recommendations on their exposure to the film character (e.g. Norman Bates in *Psycho*).

2  *Learner evaluation.* Films have been used to track educational development and performance. In this regard, responses to a film or film clip are tracked repeatedly throughout a particular course in order to assess the development of 'perceptual, conceptual and executive skills in a timely and entertaining fashion.'[5]

3  *Lecture.* A short clip shown during a lecture presentation can help to anchor teaching points and maintain learner interest.[8]

4  *Diagnosis and treatment planning.* Movies have been used to help learners to hone diagnostic and treatment formulation skills.[5] In this context, the film *Ordinary People* was shown to graduate students who were then asked to write a succession of papers based on the representation of the Jarrod family in the film. Specifically, students were asked to diagnose the main characters, assess the therapeutic methods shown in the film and develop therapeutic sessions utilizing family therapy techniques that they had already studied.

## Research overview

What is the scientific evidence to support the use of film as a teaching tool? Ber has published several articles demonstrating the effectiveness of trigger films.[29,30] In 1987, Goldman described the effect of his film-based curriculum on AIDS education.[31] More recently, Koch and Dollarhide published a qualitative assessment of their use of the movie *Good Will Hunting* in counselor education.[6] In Chapter 27 of this book, Dr Alexander presents the results of a quantitative and qualitative survey of graduate learners exposed to cinemeducation.

## Summary and caveats

A review of the literature finds well-documented use of cinema as a teaching tool for behavioral medicine and other social science education. The rationale for the use of popular cinema in education is easily demonstrated. There is mounting evidence that this is an effective mode of teaching. However, educators need to be aware that since movies are crafted primarily for entertainment purposes, they can lend themselves to stereotypical portrayals of complex human situations. Because of this, and the potential for strong emotional reactions in viewers, it is recommended that educators be actively involved in processing learner responses to cinemeducation.

## References

1.  Corneau G. Narcissus at the movies. *Hum Med* 1987; **3**: 103–9.
2.  Goode E. A rare day: the movies get mental illness right. *New York Times* 2002; **5 February**.
3.  Scorsese M. The leading man. *Rolling Stone* 2003; **922**: 89–90.
4.  Blasco PG. Literature and movies for medical students. *Fam Med* 2001; **33**: 426–8.
5.  Higgins JA, Dermer S. The use of cinema in marriage and family counselor education. *Counsel Educ Supervis* 2001; **40**: 183–93.

6.  Koch G, Dollarhide C. Using a popular film in counselor education. *Counsel Educ Supervis* 2000; **39**: 203–11.
7.  Higgins SS, Lantz JM. Nursing education: an innovative approach to using film and creative writing to teach developmental concepts to pediatric nursing students. *J Pediatr Nurs* 1997; **12**: 364–6.
8.  Alexander M, Hall M, Pettice Y. Cinemeducation: an innovative approach to teaching psychosocial medical care. *Fam Med* 1994; **26**: 430–3.
9.  Alexander M. The doctor: a seminal video for cinemeducation. *Fam Med* 2002; **34**: 92–4.
10. Karlinsky H. Doc Hollywood north. Part I. The educational application of movies in psychiatry. CPA Bulletin; www.cpa-apc.org/Publications/Archives/Bulletin/2003/february/karlinsky.asp
11. Hyler S, Moore J. Teaching psychiatry? Let Hollywood help. Suicide in the cinema. *Acad Psychiatry* 1996; **20**: 212–19.
12. Hyler S, Schanzer B. Using commercially available films to teach about borderline personality disorder. *Bull Menninger Clin* 1997; **61**: 458–68.
13. Lockhart P, Alexander M, Pettice Y, Olser R. Behavioral medicine training in postdoctoral dentist education. *J Dent Educ* 1992; **56**: 209–13.
14. Anderson D. Using feature films as tools for analysis in a psychology and law course. *Teach Psychol* 1992; **19**: 155–8.
15. Alexander M, Waxman D. Cinemeducation: teaching family systems through the movies. *Fam Syst Health* 2000; **18**: 455–66.
16. Maynard P. Teaching family therapy theory: do something different. *J Am Fam Ther* 1996; **24**: 195–204.
17. Alexander M. Cinemeducation: an innovative approach to teaching multi-cultural diversity in medicine. *Ann Behav Sci Med Educ* 1995; **2**: 23–8.
18. Pinterits EJ, Atkinson DR. The diversity video forum: an adjunct to diversity sensitivity training in the classroom. *Counsel Educ Supervis* 1998; **37**: 203–16.
19. Tyler LM, Reynolds T. Using feature films to teach group counseling. *J Specialists Group Work* 1998; **23**: 7–21.
20. Chambliss C, Magatis G. *Videotapes for Use in Teaching Psychopathology.* Lanham, MD: ERIC Document Reproduction Service, 1996.
21. Gabbard GO, Gabbard K. *Psychiatry and the Cinema* (2e). Washington, DC: American Psychiatric Press Inc, 1999.
22. Wedding D, Boyd MA. *Movies and Mental Illness: using films to understand psychopathology.* Boston, MA: McGraw-Hill College, 1999 (out of print).
23. Robinson DJ. *Reel Psychiatry: movie portrayals of psychiatric conditions.* London: Rapid Psychler Press, 2003.
24. Koren G. Awakenings: using a popular movie to teach clinical pharmacology. *Clin Pharmacol Ther* 1993; **53**: 3–5.
25. Hesley JW, Hesley JG. *Rent Two Films and Let's Talk in the Morning* (2e). New York: John Wiley and Sons, 2001.
26. Dermer SB, Hutchings JB. Utilizing movies in family therapy: applications for individuals, couples and families. *Am J Fam Ther* 2000; **28**: 163–80.
27. Peterson LW. *A Therapist's Guide to the Horse Whisperer: intervening with parents of traumatized children.* Grosse Pointe, MI: The National Institute for Trauma and Loss in Children, 2003.
28. Zazulak J. Let Hollywood help you teach. *SOT Newsletter* 2002; **10**; www.cfpc.ca/English/cfpc/education/section20of20teachers/newsletter/volume201020number201/default.asp?s=1
29. Ber R. Teaching professionalism with the art of trigger questions. *Med Teach* 2003; **24**: 528–31.

30. Ber R. Twenty years of experience using trigger films as a teaching tool. *Acad Med* 2001; **76**: 656–8.
31. Goldman JD. An elective seminar to teach first year medical students the social and medical aspects of AIDS. *J Med Educ* 1987; **62**: 557–61.

# Chapter 2

# Film and narrative medicine: cinemeducation and the development of narrative competence

*Vincent MB Silenzio, Craig A Irvine, Robert E Sember and Bertie E Bregman*

## Overview

The use of films, in whole or in part, has been an important but under-utilized part of medical education for most of the past century. The field of narrative medicine has developed with the recognition of the central role of narrative competence for technically appropriate, socially acceptable and culturally sensitive clinical practice. Essentially, universal appreciation of film and video, coupled with relative efficiencies in time, implies that narrative film studies offer many advantages over more traditional medical humanities approaches. We here describe a basic curriculum in narrative film studies to develop narrative competence for medical personnel, and we provide a brief introduction to the emerging field of narrative medicine.

> *I am kino-eye, I am a mechanical eye. I, a machine, show you the world as only I can see it . . . . My path leads to the creation of a fresh perception of the world I decipher in a new way, a world unknown to you.*[1]

While ushering in the fully modern notion of the movie camera as the unflinching, all-seeing eye, Dziga Vertov, one of the early Soviet intellectuals so centrally important to the first century of film, expresses one of the key metaphors of our age. He also touches on some of our most pressing questions about the relationship between the 'real' world and the representations which we create of that world. From the moment of its inception, the cinema has helped in exciting new ways to raise the very same issues of reality and representation that have occupied human thought for millennia. Concern with these issues is no less relevant for medicine, and poses an ongoing challenge – and opportunity – for medical education.

There are three basic ways in which films have been used in medical education. The first has been in the explicit instructional realm, and these types of film have been a part of medical education for decades. The second has been in the use of films to grapple with the range of experiences possible in medical education,[2] training or practice,[3] and to reflect on the biopsychosocial roles of medical personnel in society. The cinema becomes a mirror into which medical practitioners may peer to see how others see them, or how they and others experience illness and the passages of life. As in a Hall of Mirrors, these reflections may be distorted in interesting and provocative ways that stretch the viewer's perceptions and lead to novel insights – as well as to misperception-informed conclusions about the 'real' world. Dealing with the possibilities of the former and the dangers of the latter has occupied much of the thought and energy of medical humanities educators. This approach represents the principal form of cinemeducation discussed in the remainder of this book.

A third use of film in medical education has been to utilize the study of the cinematic arts as a tool to understand the social, economic, political and scientific dimensions of clinical and public health practice. Narrative analysis and film studies, in this third approach, become a kind of basic science for medical learners to master. A foundation in these disciplines serves to provide the student with tools to understand and address the narrative structure of patient and provider experiences, improve communication skills, and improve clinical and diagnostic reasoning. This toolset has been referred to as *narrative competence*,[4] and refers to the ability of clinicians to competently understand and respond to the complexity of the narrative situations with which they are commonly confronted. Appreciating the lived experiences of physicians, patients, families, communities and societies from the narrative perspective (i.e. as stories amenable to the techniques of narrative analysis and critique) affords the opportunity to nurture skills in this dimension of clinical practice.[5–7]

# Narrative medicine: what and why?

Medical humanities have proved useful in addressing the myriad experiences of clinical practice. The humanities provide physicians and others with a set of tools with which to organize and understand their complex perceptions confronted in the clinical trenches. Within the medical humanities, interest has grown in the study of narrative theory and its clinical applications.[4] Writers such as Hunter have emphasized that clinical reason is a basic application of narrative knowledge,[8] namely the forms of knowledge that are used to understand the meaning and significance of stories through cognitive, symbolic and affective means.

The application of narrative methods in the medical humanities has been dubbed *narrative medicine*.[9] Narrative medicine refers to a mode of clinical practice in which the clinician is competent to 'recognize, interpret, and be moved to action by the predicaments of others.'[9] At the core of healing or therapeutic engagement has been the inter-subjective experience of the healer and others in ever-widening social circles. When authentic, this engagement is transformative for all participants. The 'narrative' is the story, typically constructed at first singly by the individual, and then socially with his or her family and community, and with the clinician. This process of selecting relevant details, placing them in relation to one another in time and importance, and projecting possible future expectations has been called *therapeutic emplotment*.[10] It is this construction of 'plot' that helps us understand what has come before, what is occurring now and what is likely to happen in the future. From this perspective, 'illness' is the disruption of the plot line as previously expected, and therapeutic engagement is the attempt by socially sanctioned healers to help renarrate and rewrite the story. This process is conducted through the use of narrative storytelling, just as the communication of this story between and by professionals relies upon constructions of narrative.

The study of film and documentary offers learners the opportunity to broaden their appreciation of cinema and develop narrative competence, and provides educators with a potent tool to increase learners' sensitivity to patient, family, community, cultural and personal concerns. Adapting the schema proposed by Charon,[4] the types of narrative situation commonly encountered in family practice include *family/patient–physician, physician–self, physician–colleagues* and *physician–community/society*.[11] Through mastery of basic narrative analytic techniques and exploration of the creative processes involved in documenting medical experience, medical students and practitioners may gain important competencies in narrative that foster patient-centered, compassionate, empathic care in each of these narrative situations.

## Why cinema for narrative medicine?

As part of the renewed interest in narrative studies in medicine, there has been growing interest in film as an educational vehicle to address important educational objectives with regard to knowledge, skills or attitudes.[11] Film studies can overcome many of the limitations of more traditional forms of medical humanities curricula, and focus attention on the narrative structure of medical experience. Although many learners may find advanced analyses of poetry, prose or other arts to be dauntingly unfamiliar territory, these same learners, as the products of a modern, visual culture, commonly possess untapped critical abilities in cinema that can be developed more fully. This nascent, widespread aesthetic appreciation of film also offers an important advantage over existing medical humanities curricular models in terms of time efficiency. Films can be experienced with immediacy, permitting a broad experience that would otherwise be difficult to achieve in the usually limited time available, and almost every learner possesses enough critical capacity to gain meaningful insights through the experience of watching films.

We have developed an approach to formal studies in film and narrative analysis in medical education and training using a discussion series in Medical Cinema Studies. The fundamental approach is described here, and it can be adapted to a variety of residency training and medical education settings. Each session of the discussion series provides participants with one or more basic critical skills from narrative film theory in an effort to promote narrative competence more broadly, and strives to facilitate learners' appreciation of the applicability of these insights to clinical practice. Participants also examine cinema's potential in professional education, training and socialization.

Each session centers discussion around a single film, using either familiar or relatively unknown films that have been selected to help to stimulate participant interest. The crucial intellectual point of departure for us has been that the films selected for study remain explicitly *non*-medical in plot or topic, freeing learners to focus on the concepts rather than on the 'medical' details of the film. As is shown by the range of films listed in the filmography below, this has provided the freedom to select from an impressive array of films, from blockbusters to classics to *avant-garde* experiments. Each film is used to exemplify one or more specific cinematic issues examined in the context of medical thought and practice. Films are screened in whole or in part prior to the session in order to stimulate discussion relevant to the goals and objectives of each educational interaction. For more straightforward knowledge or skills objectives, well-selected clips may suffice to stimulate discussion. However, in our experience, attitudinal objectives have been easier to address through the use of full films, or even through screening multiple films at one time.

Learners are first introduced to basic narrative forms and structures. If desired, subsequent sessions can progress to an examination of the ways in which culture, ideology and historical circumstance influence the telling or reception of stories in often invisible and unconscious ways. Throughout the discussions, learners are repeatedly asked to examine the issues implied in our contemporary vision of the physician as one who performs the roles of both scientist and humanist. Do we experience reality differently in the cinematic age – that is, have our eyes indeed become cameras? What is the origin of the meaning in what we see? If necessary, how do we edit or write visual reality into structures of meaning that enable us to influence or perhaps even heal reality? Building upon the aesthetic competence that they already possess and depending on the time available, participants learn to articulate their analyses in new and more nuanced ways.[12]

The curriculum addresses six key areas of narrative studies in order to explore the direct implications of narrative studies in medicine. When further materials for self-directed learning are desired, readings drawn from standard film studies textbooks[13–16] and the medical literature[17–19] are readily available for each area.

## Narrative and representation: from Aristotle to postmodernism

*Fabula*? *Syuzhet*? Call them *story* and *plot* instead, if you prefer. But introducing basic concepts and jargon from cinema studies allows learners to begin to explore how the structure of narrative and concepts such as *point of view (POV), perspective* and others explored in subsequent discussions can help them to understand lived experiences.

## Mythology, fairy tales and other true stories: archetypal narratives in film and medicine

Writers such as Propp and Grimas have expanded our understanding of myths and other forms of narrative in a culture that both sustains and creates its own symbols and metaphors. In what way have movies become the myths of our times? What are the myths in medical practice, and can medical encounters and stories be analyzed using similar approaches?

## Cultural mirror or mold: authorship, *auteurs* and social production

What social processes are necessary for stories to be produced, and how does the structure of the 'Dream Factory' influence how these stories are told, what is included and what is left out? Is there an analogous social production process in clinical medicine? Who is the author of a story? Is it the same person as the narrator? Who is the 'author' of a film, or of a medical history? How does the range of possible answers to these questions influence the experiences of health or disease and the processes of caring and healing?

## Ideology in film and at the bedside: thinking inside the box

What is *ideology*, and what possible role could such a thing play in the coolly objective, purely scientific world of medicine? The insights gained from analyzing ideology in films can be used to delve deeply into this question.

## Reel realism: re-presenting reality in film – lessons for medicine

Realism is a deceptively simple concept in film and other representations. What is the 'suspension of disbelief' that is so central to the experience of the 'real' in film? How does this relate to the creation and sharing of medical narratives? If issues of ideology do indeed color all perception, what is the relationship between truth, reality and representation?

## From prose to poetry: documentary, experimental and other cinemas

Feature films typically follow conventional narrative rules. So-called 'non-narrative' films offer the chance to reflect on how we strive to make sense of the world we see before us, even if this is experienced outside the conventional rules. We each see the same film, yet we each see it differently. We appreciate the same experiences, yet we experience them quite distinctly. Of what use are these insights to clinicians? What can this tell us about the practice of medicine?

## Going further

There are simple strategies that can be employed to allow students and residents to go further or to explore the practical implications of what they have learned. One such approach would be to include a production component, through which learners produce a short video project exploring themes arising during the course. Such production experiences, once prohibitively expensive and time-consuming, are now practical thanks to advances in low-cost digital video production and the creation of easily mastered software such as iMovie.[20] Advanced curricula can further emphasize the explicit connections between the representation of reality in documentary cinema and in medicine. Coles and others have highlighted this relationship, arguing that documentary work may be construed as a narrative constructed by the observer that is ultimately meant not simply to represent 'reality' but to interpret it.[21–24] Learners have the opportunity to conceptualize, film, edit and produce their own production projects, and to learn the differences between fictional and documentary films. Although they may never directly work in documentary film production again, participants gain insights into the collaborative processes involved and the major ethical issues in documentary work. Learners can explore lessons from film and documentary for their clinical work and make the connections between patients' and families' experiences of health and illness as narrative phenomena.

## Summary

Narrative medicine and film studies represent an important way in which cinemeducation remains at the forefront of medical education. Films that do not explicitly deal with medical concerns ideally challenge learners to consider how to generalize lessons in narrative to medical situations. In addition to using selected clips to demonstrate key educational points, screening full-length films may be an excellent way to stimulate discussion and begin to address attitudinal learning objectives. The filmography below lists the films that we have used in our work with medical students and residents over the past four years, and indicates how we have used the films.

## Selected filmography

*Note*: There are no explicitly 'medical' films listed here. The basic premise of using film studies to promote narrative competence is that gaining knowledge and skills in narrative analysis is key to fostering narrative competencies for medical learners. Using important contemporary and historical films gives learners the opportunity to focus on the basics of narrative analysis without getting bogged down in questions of medical 'accuracy' or verisimilitude, and offers educators an opportunity to approach attitudinal learning through the careful selection of psychological, social, economic, political, moral, ethical and philosophical areas for discussion.

◆ *Being John Malkovich* (1999, 112 min, USA, Director Spike Jonze). Ever wonder what it would be like to get inside the head of a famous actor? Let's just say you'll eventually end up at the side of the road on a New Jersey turnpike exit ramp. Existential questions have arguably never had more interesting answers.

◆ *Casablanca* (1942, 102 min, USA, Director Michael Curtiz). The love between Bogart and Bergman is so intense that it is pointless to propose any resistance. Unless, of course, that resistance is led by Victor Laszlo. Often forgotten these days is the fact that the USA was ostensibly *neutral* at the time when this film was made. Casablanca remains an awe-inspiring example of what the Dream Factory of Hollywood's Golden Era could produce, when highly polished pictures were being pumped out at a rate of one or more per week by each of the studios. Casablanca is brimming over with memorable lines and scenes, such as the response to the Gestapo Major's question of whether Rick (Bogart) could imagine the Germans in his native New York, when Bogie utters the memorable deadpan 'There are certain sections of New York, Major, that I wouldn't advise you to try to invade.'

◆ *Citizen Kane* (1941, 119 min, USA, Director Orson Welles). Xanadu knew Kubla Khan and Citizen Kane. Welles' thinly veiled biopic of William Randolph Hearst embroiled both of these powerful and brilliant men in one of the epic battles of Hollywood history. Astonishingly, Welles produced this technical masterpiece as his first movie.

◆ *Crouching Tiger, Hidden Dragon* (2000, 120 min, USA, Director Ang Lee). What do you get when Ang Lee (*Sense and Sensibility, The Wedding Banquet, The Ice Storm* and *Eat, Drink, Man, Woman*) decides to make a homage film to the martial arts masterpieces of Hong Kong cinema? The anwer is an awesomely masterful action-flick-as-magical-love-story. There are few better examples of movies as modern myth making than this non-stop, lyrical reflection on love, honor and human potential.

◆ *La Dolce Vita* (1960, 167 min, Italy, Director Federico Fellini). The term *paparazzi* was coined and an entire aesthetic gained a firm grip on the imagination of the Western world based on this simple, eloquent exploration of the vapid nature of twentieth-century fame.

◆ *Manhattan Murder Mystery* (1994, 104 min, USA, Director Woody Allen). It is not an exaggeration to say that any film by Woody Allen could be used to address just about any issue in narrative medicine. For example, few works of art have captured the ethnic diversity of family life with such agile grace as the dinner scene of *Annie Hall*. Murder and mayhem reign supreme in this comic thriller starring Alan Alda, Mia Farrow, Angelica Huston, Woody Allen and, of course, Allen's beloved Manhattan.

◆ *The Matrix* (1999, 136 min, USA, Directors Andy and Larry Wachowski). *The Matrix* was not only a smash box-office success, but also has arguably had an immeasurable impact on the art of film making ever since. The Wachowski brothers indulge their comic book/animé/Hong Kong fetishes, and produce an astonishingly accessible tale of the limits of reason and perception.

◆ *Rashomon* (1950, 88 min, Japan, Director Akira Kurosawa). At the symbolic gates of a ruined Japanese city in the Middle Ages, a group of people brought together by the need to escape a storm lead one of the most intriguing explorations of narrative truth ever to be committed to film. *Rashomon* is the film that catapulted the great director of *Seven Samurai* and *Ran* to international stardom.

◆ *Rear Window* (1954, 112 min, USA, Director Alfred Hitchcock). Cooped up in his Greenwich Village apartment while recovering from a broken leg, Jimmy Stewart plays a stir-crazy photographer who bides his time staring through his lens at his neighbors across the courtyard. But when he notices one of his neighbors is missing, is it the summer heat getting to him, or is it a real Greenwich Village murder mystery? Hitchcock's reflections on the thin line between movie going and voyeurism, along with stellar performances by Grace Kelly and Thelma Ritter, make this a mystery worth contemplating.

◆ *Rome, Open City* (1946, 100 min, Italy, Director Roberto Rossellini). The effects of the neorealist movement in film are being felt to this day. Shot on the streets of Rome while the front line was only a handful of miles to the north, this gritty tale of death and resistance stays with you long after it is over. That these are mostly non-professionals working in real settings (the complete opposite of the Hollywood studio system), and that the results are so impressive, helps to explain why the brief neorealist movement was so influential in the history of film.

◆ *The Seventh Seal* (1957, 92 min, Sweden, Director Ingmar Bergman). Max von Sydow stars as a returning Crusader Knight who battles Death in a fateful game of chess. A plague-racked, spiritually bankrupt, medieval Sweden serves as the backdrop to this musing on faith, family and redemption.

◆ *The Shining* (1980, 119/140 min, GB, Director Stanley Kubrick). Cooped up in his Winter Palace, Jack Nicholson slowly begins to lose his grip. Shelly Duvall and Danny Lloyd are his co-cooped-up wife and son, but when things start turning weird, it's déjà vu all over again. This contains some of the most important filmed sequences of the late twentieth century, as Kubrick brings us along visually and aurally on Jack's downhill whirlwind ride. It is a scary movie.

◆ *Silverlake Life: the View from Here* (1993, Directors Peter Friedman and Tom Joslin). Seeing is believing. That is the fundamental tenet of modern medical knowledge. In medical education and training, students are socialized to a visual knowledge of the human body, and come to privilege visual over all other metaphors in conceptualizing the mysteries of life. Other professionals who do the same include film and video artists. *Silverlake Life* offers a heart-rending experience of one man's struggle with the loss of vision and life, and the process of representing his own death through visual media.

◆ *South Park: Bigger, Longer, and Uncut* (1999, Director Trey Parker). Leave it to an animated feature to explicitly shatter our false sense of security that overtly ideological films have somehow been relegated to the dustbin of history. After all, how would it be possible to make Saddam Hussein the gay lover of Satan without a libel suit, if not for the fact that he is the quintessential enemy of the Brave New World Order? But there is more here than simple vilification of the bad guys. Swimming amidst the bath water of toilet humor is a subtle critique of the role that the media plays in our lives, and the types of mediated violence that we deem acceptable and unacceptable.

◆ *Star Wars* (1976, USA, Director George Lucas). The battle between good and evil, and all shades of moral value in between, has at least been ongoing since long, long ago in a galaxy far, far away. It is apparently also continuing to rage in contemporary film. In one of the final scenes of this film, Lucas pays tribute to a sequence of a solemn ceremony taken directly from the Nazi propaganda masterpiece *Triumph des Willens* (see below).

◆ *Le Locataire* (*The Tenant*, 1976, 125 min, USA/France, Director Roman Polanski). The fact that his wife, the actress Sharon Tate, had long since been the victim of one of the most famous murders in American history gives Polanski's film musings on madness an added dimension of experience that few directors can match. The analytic possibilities of his film *Rosemary's Baby* alone could occupy an interestingly lengthy discussion. In *The Tenant*, Polanski leads us through the slow and steady descent into unreason that one risks by 'harmlessly' appropriating the coveted Parisian apartment of a dying woman.

◆ *Trainspotting* (1998, 94 min, Scotland, Director Danny Boyle). 'Choose life. Choose a job. Choose a starter home. Choose dental insurance, leisurewear and matching luggage. Choose your future. But why would anyone want to do a thing like that?' Few things challenge our notion of selfhood and integrity more than encounters with individuals and communities that utterly refuse to share our values. Fortunately, both film and clinical practice afford us unlimited opportunities to encounter these challenges. This film challenges us to confront the possibility that the best of us will learn and grow from these experiences, while others will ossify into phlegmatic technocrats, biding our time until the glorious days of cashing in our retirement plans.

◆ *Triumph des Willens* (*Triumph of the Will*, 1934, Director Leni Riefenstahl). This film is stunning in every sense of the word. Documenting the Sixth Nazi Party Congress in Nuremburg, Riefenstahl created the most artful, visually rich and cunning propaganda film of all time. Although she was never convicted of war crimes, her career was ironically destroyed by the unfortunate greatness of her Nazi-era successes. Nonetheless, Riefenstahl's directorial work has exerted a profound influence on cinema ever since. In *Olympiad*, documenting the 1936 Berlin Olympics, she literally established how sports have been covered ever since. Riefenstahl remains one of the greatest and most controversial directors of the twentieth century.

◆ *Un Chien Andalou* (1929, 90 min, France, Director Luis Buñuel). Out of the minds of Buñuel and Salvador Dali comes a truly surreal experience. The eye-cutting sequence is understandably one of the most (in)famous in all of cinema.

## References

1. Vertov D, Michelson A. *Kino-Eye: the writings of Dziga Vertov.* Berkeley, CA: University of California Press, 1984.
2. Conn JJ. What can clinical teachers learn from *Harry Potter and the Philosopher's Stone? Med Educ* 2002; **36**: 1176–81.
3. Elder NC, Schwarzer A. Using the cinema to understand the family of the alcoholic. *Fam Med* 2002; **34**: 426–7.
4. Charon R. The patient–physician relationship. Narrative medicine: a model for empathy, reflection, profession and trust. *JAMA* 2001; **286**: 1897–902.
5. Mattingly C, Garro L. *Narrative and the Cultural Construction of Illness and Healing.* Berkeley, CA: University of California Press, 2000.
6. Mattingly C. *Healing Dramas and Clinical Plots: the narrative structure of experience.* Cambridge, NY: Cambridge University Press, 1998.
7. Greenhalgh T, Hurwitz B. *Narrative-Based Medicine: dialogue and discourse in clinical practice.* London: BMJ Books, 1998.
8. Hunter KM. Narrative, literature and the clinical exercise of practical reason. *J Med Philos* 1996; **21**: 303–20.
9. Charon R. Narrative medicine: form, function and ethics. *Ann Intern Med* 2001; **134**: 83–7.
10. Mattingly C. The concept of therapeutic 'emplotment.' *Soc Sci Med* 1994; **38**: 811–22.
11. Silenzio V. Things my VCR never told me: film studies and narrative medicine. *STFM Messenger* 2002; **22**: 2–3.
12. Silenzio VMB, Irvine CA, Bregman BE, Sember R. *Kino-Pravda: improving clinical communication skills through a curriculum in medical cinema studies.* Predoctoral Education Conference Presentation. Long Beach, CA: Society of Teachers of Family Medicine, 2001.
13. Bordwell D, Thompson K. *Film Art: an introduction* (6e). New York: McGraw-Hill Companies, 2001.
14. Bordwell D. *The McGraw-Hill Film Viewer's Guide.* New York: McGraw-Hill Companies, 2001.
15. Corrigan T. *A Short Guide to Writing About Film* (3e). New York: Longman, 1998.
16. Monaco J. *How to Read a Film: the world of movies, media and multimedia. Language, history, theory* (3e). New York: Oxford University Press, 2000.
17. Crawford TH. Visual knowledge in medicine and popular film. *Lit Med* 1998; **17**: 24–44.
18. Shapiro JF. Atomic bomb cinema: illness, suffering and the apocalyptic narrative. *Lit Med* 1998; **17**: 126–48.
19. Dans PE. The temple of healing: reflections from a physician at the movies. *Lit Med* 1998; 17: 114–25.
20. Rubin M. Apple Training Series: iLife04. Berkeley, CA: Peachpit Press, 2004.
21. Nichols B. *Introduction to Documentary.* Bloomington, IN: Indiana University Press, 2001.
22. Coles R. *Doing Documentary Work.* New York: Oxford University Press, 1997.

23. Nichols B. *Representing Reality: issues and concepts in documentary*. Bloomington, IN: Indiana University Press, 1991.
24. Barnouw E. *Documentary: a history of the non-fiction film* (2e). New York: Oxford University Press, 1993.

# Part II

## The individual and family life cycle

# Chapter 3

# Child and adolescent development

*Anna Pavlov*

Family physicians provide healthcare to people throughout their lifespan. Family doctors are at the forefront as individuals contemplate having children. Likewise, they provide prenatal, postnatal, pediatric and adolescent care. They are often the first healthcare providers to whom parents come for advice and to voice concerns about their children. For all of these reasons, family physicians are in a key position to provide information, anticipatory guidance, reassurance, counseling and referral for individuals and families who need support and assistance with various developmental challenges and family circumstances.

## Caring for a baby's needs

◆ *Baby Boom* (Diane Keaton). This film portrays the adjustment of a highly successful and driven businesswoman, JC (Diane Keaton), who is suddenly thrust into the role of mother when a distant cousin dies and she is the only relative available to look after her baby girl.

a (0:17:09–0:24:13). JC juggles the handling of the immediate needs of baby Elizabeth. She struggles to change her diaper and attempts to feed the baby 'adult' food. She and her partner are high functioning in many areas, but are not experienced in 'baby basics.'

1  What are some of the 'baby basics' revealed in this clip?
2  How equipped do you feel to respond to a new parent's questions? What areas remain difficult?
3  How do you approach what appears to be an 'overanxious mother'?
4  How would you be able to tell/know when a parent needs to be referred for counseling/parenting issues?

b (0:25:43–0:28:34). The baby has a high fever and JC is trying to figure out what to do. She orders some baby medical supplies that are delivered along with a bottle of Valium for herself.

1  How do you respond when a parent telephones you concerned about their baby?
2  What recommendations do you offer parents regarding their own care and well-being?
3  What would you say/do if a parent acknowledges 'losing it' with their child and/or is afraid that they will hurt the child?

# Discipline

## Child testing limits

◆ *Kramer vs Kramer* (Dustin Hoffman, Meryl Streep, Justin Henry). This film depicts the struggles facing a successful marketing executive who suddenly becomes a single parent of a 6-year-old son after his wife leaves him. Ted Kramer (Dustin Hoffman) eventually adjusts to the situation and enjoys raising his son, Billy (Justin Henry), only to face a custody stand-off with his ex-wife (Meryl Streep).

a (0:35:18–0:38:50). In this clip, Ted is setting limits on his son's TV time. At dinner Billy picks at his food. He tests his father's limits by ignoring repeated warnings to eat his food and not leave the table to go for ice cream.

1 How would you respond to a situation in the exam room where a parent is not setting limits on their child?
2 Given what you saw in this clip, what advice would you have for Ted about how he might have handled this situation better?
3 What advice would you give a parent who is complaining about a 'picky eater'?
4 How equipped do you feel to respond to parents' questions about their children's behavior? For those who don't have their own children, how can you become more confident in giving advice to parents? What experiences/readings could assist you?

## Physical punishment

◆ *Dennis the Menace* (Walter Matthau, Mason Gamble, Joan Plowright, Christopher Lloyd, Lea Thompson, Paul Winfield). This film, based on the comic strip, depicts 5-year-old Dennis as a bright, well-meaning and precocious child. His antics always seem to impact negatively on his retired neighbor, Mr Wilson.

a (0:8:40–0:09:42). Dennis' father apologizes to Mr Wilson. Mr Wilson tells him that Dennis is driving him 'nuts.' Mr Mitchell says that he will talk to Dennis, while Mr Wilson suggests physical punishment.

b (0:13:10–0:13:36). Dennis does not want to spend his days at Margaret's house. His mother drags him out of the car on to the sidewalk, and into the house.

1 What is the American Academy of Pediatrics' stance on the use of physical punishment?
2 How do you counsel parents with regard to punishment? What are your feelings/values with regard to physical punishment? Is talking to a child about problem behavior always appropriate?
3 Suggest some alternative approaches for the behaviors depicted.
4 What are your views in general about the best way to discipline a child?
5 What would you do if a parent spanked their child in the exam room?

## 'Time out' for misbehavior

◆ *Dennis the Menace* (Walter Matthau, Mason Gamble, Joan Plowright, Christopher Lloyd, Lea Thompson, Paul Winfield). See previous section on physical punishment for movie description.

a (0:07:17–0:08:00). Dennis' mother asks if he used his slingshot to shoot an aspirin into Mr Wilson's mouth. His father takes the slingshot from him and tells Dennis to go and sit in the corner until he is sorry. Dennis' mother informs her husband that she has to leave.

1   How equipped do you feel to respond to parents' questions about their children's behavior? For those who don't have their own children, how can you become more confident in giving advice to parents? What experiences/ readings can you seek out to assist you?
2   What instructions would you give a parent on how to use 'time out' to manage behavior problems?
3   What are some common misuses of 'time out' (e.g. sending the child to their room and keeping the child in 'time out' for too long)?

## Ingredients of a good parent

◆ *Kramer vs Kramer* (Dustin Hoffman, Meryl Streep, Justin Henry). See previous section on child testing limits for movie description.

a (1:28:00–1:28:55). While testifying in the custody hearing with his ex-wife, Ted describes what it takes to be a good parent (constancy and listening even when you can't listen anymore).

1   In what ways can you reinforce good parenting skills and support parents? What can you say?
2   What would you do if a parent confessed to you that they struck their child in a moment of anger?
3   What would you do if a nurse told you that she noticed a parent being 'rough with a child'?

# Developmental issues

## 'Magical thinking'

◆ *Kramer vs Kramer* (Dustin Hoffman, Meryl Streep, Justin Henry). See previous section on child testing limits/discipline for movie description.

a (0:39:00–0:42:10). Ted checks on Billy, who is now asleep. He awakens and they each apologize for the unpleasantness at dinnertime. Billy worries that his dad, too, may go away. He wonders if his mother left because of something he did: 'Did mom leave because I was bad?'

1   Billy is demonstrating the concept of 'magical thinking.' Solicit audience awareness of the meaning of this term, and then provide a definition.

2 What are some medical situations in which a child may engage in 'magical thinking'?

3 What are the best ways for divorcing parents to talk to their children about their reasons for separating?

## Self-esteem/childhood teasing

◆ *About a Boy* (Hugh Grant, Rachel Weisz, Toni Collette). Will (Hugh Grant) is the perennial bachelor who believes that 'every man is an island unto himself'. He invents an imaginary son in order to meet attractive single mothers. In the process he develops a unique friendship with 12-year-old called Marcus, who struggles as the son of a very depressed mother.

a (0:01:17–0:02:16). We hear Marcus' thoughts of feeling as if he doesn't fit in, either at his old school or at his new one.

b (0:11:31–0:12:32). Boys at school are kicking a ball at Marcus. Two boys tell him that they do not want him hanging around them anymore because other boys are harassing them. One boy tells Marcus that everyone thinks he is weird. Marcus comments to himself that he is having a bad time at home and at school.

1 What are the effects of childhood teasing/harassment?

2 How would you counsel a parent who sought your advice about what to do in this situation?

3 In what ways can maternal depression impact a child?

### Adolescent individuation/rebellion

◆ *Life as a House* (Kevin Kline, Kristin Scott Thomas, Hayden Christensen). George (Kevin Kline), an architect, uses the construction of a new house as a way of rebuilding his life, including his relationship with his troubled teenage son, once he learns that he is dying. Sam (Hayden Christensen) displays adolescent rebellion, sexual identity issues and anger toward his parents, who are divorced. He gets to know his father by participating in the construction of his new house.

a (0:05:50–0:06:45). The blended family is having breakfast. Sam's mother asks her husband to talk with her son (his stepson). Sam is confronted about his eye make-up, and behind his back a younger stepbrother calls him a 'queer.' The stepbrother then justifies his remark by saying 'Dad did it first.'

b (0:09:05–0:11:50). Sam's father, George, stops by the house and is talking with his ex-wife in the kitchen. He asks why she allowed Sam to pierce his chin. Her response is 'What kind of a mother can't stand her own son?' George attempts to break down the barriers between himself and his son by going into Sam's room any way that he can. Sam then yells at his parents for invading his space.

1 What approach would you take with a parent who complained of having no control over their teenager? How would you counsel parents who disapproved of their teenager's clothes, make-up, etc.?

2 How would you handle a situation where a parent brought a teenager in to see you and demanded drug testing?

3  How do you approach interviewing an adolescent?
4  Review the BIHEADSS mnemonic (**B**ody Image, **H**ome, **E**ducation, **A**ctivities, **D**rug use, **S**exual practices, **S**uicidal ideation).

# Attention deficit hyperactivity disorder (AD/HD)

◆ *Dennis the Menace* (Walter Matthau, Mason Gamble, Joan Plowright, Christopher Lloyd, Lea Thompson, Paul Winfield). See previous section on physical punishment for movie description.

a  (0:35:08–0:39:00). Dennis goes to the Wilsons' home with a card of apology for Mr Wilson. He asks Mrs Wilson if he can go upstairs to place the card near Mr Wilson. Dennis talks excessively, disclosing inappropriate details about his family life and his struggle with impulsivity. He cannot resist playing with Mr Wilson's dentures and he breaks them. We see Dennis' solution to repairing the dentures just prior to Mr Wilson awakening for an important photograph.

b  (0:47:15–0:47:48). Dennis is being looked after by the Wilsons while his parents are away. While he is in the bathtub he is in constant motion as he twirls round and round singing and splashing water onto the bathroom floor.

1  Which symptoms of AD/HD do we see in these two clips?
2  What are the DSM-IV diagnostic criteria for AD/HD?
3  What are the American Academy of Pediatrics' practice guidelines for assessing AD/HD?
4  What conditions can mimic AD/HD and/or coexist with it?

c  (0:41:46–0:42:45). Dennis' parents are calling everyone they know who might be able to care for their son while they are away. We see them systematically going through their phone book with no results as we view each prospective sitter's responses to the thought of spending time with Dennis.

1  What are some of the challenges of parenting a child with AD/HD?
2  How would you explain AD/HD to a parent? What would you say to the child?
3  How would you respond to a parent's hesitation about initiating a trial of psychostimulant medication?
4  How would you respond to a parent's concern that being on psychostimulant medication could cause substance abuse?

# Adjustment to divorce

◆ *Kramer vs Kramer* (Dustin Hoffman, Meryl Streep, Justin Henry). See previous section on child testing limits/discipline for movie description.

a  (0:11:55–0:12:50). Joanna informs Ted that she is leaving the marriage. She reviews what she has taken care of and walks out the door.

b  (0:18:20–0:20:02). Ted's boss confronts him about his ability to do his work while single-parenting his son.

c  (0:22:15–0:25:02). Ted reads Billy a letter from his mother in which she explains her absence. At one point Billy can listen no more and turns up the volume on his cartoon program.

1  If a parent expressed concern to you about the impact of divorce on their child, what advice would you give them?
2  For those of you who are parents, what is it like for you to juggle your various roles?

## Special situations

### Parent involvement during an acute medical crisis

◆ *Kramer vs Kramer* (Dustin Hoffman, Meryl Streep, Justin Henry). See previous section on child testing limits/discipline for movie description.

a  (0:47:24–0:49:45). Billy gets hurt on the jungle gym. Ted insists on remaining with his son in the emergency room while he is being treated.

1  What do you think of the physician's interaction with a distressed father?
2  How do you handle situations in the emergency room that involve parents and young children?

### Malingering

◆ *E.T. The Extra Terrestrial* (Henry Thomas, Robert MacNaughton, Drew Barrymore). This famous movie tells the story of an alien who is befriended by a young boy named Elliott (Henry Thomas).

a  (0:25:24–0:27:15). In this scene, Elliott fakes a high temperature.

1  How common is malingering among children? Why might children engage in this behavior? How would you counsel parents whose children routinely feign illness to avoid school?
2  How is malingering different from factitious disorder?
3  Have you encountered malingering among adult patients? How have you dealt with this problem? How does it make you feel when you discover that patients are exaggerating claims of illness for secondary gain?

### The child/teenager in foster care/parent incarcerated

◆ *White Oleander* (Michelle Pfeiffer, Renee Zellweger, Alison Lohman). Astrid (Alison Lohman) is placed in multiple foster homes and residential programs after her mother (Michelle Pfeiffer) is incarcerated for the murder of her boyfriend. Astrid's personality-disordered mother manipulates and undermines any and all attachments that she forms. This pattern continues until the end of the film, when her mother takes responsibility for her own murderous behavior and does not allow Astrid to testify on her behalf.

a  (0:11:40–0:16:44). Children's Services arrive to pick up Astrid. They tell her that her mother has been arrested. She watches in the courtroom as her mother is sentenced. Astrid's social worker drives her to her first foster home, where she is introduced to the foster family.

1   What reactions/emotions did you have when viewing Astrid being taken from her home and placed in foster care?
2   What are some of the unique issues specific to foster children? How can we assist such children?

b   (1:33:44–1:38:10). Astrid confronts her mother about a woman she vaguely remembers from the past who was a part of her life. Her mother describes having felt ill-prepared to be a mother, trapped by her baby's continuous needs and fearing she would be abusive towards her. She tells Astrid that one day she left her with a neighbor so that she could get a break, and she ended up being gone for over a year.

1   What feelings does this clip bring up? Do you feel sympathetic towards the mother? Why or why not? What other clinical situations might trigger similar feelings? For example, what do you notice about how you feel towards/interact with a mother who abused drugs during pregnancy and whose baby is in the neonatal intensive-care unit?
2   How would you respond to a new mother who voiced doubts about being a mother?

## Death of a parent

◆   *Life as a House* (Kevin Kline, Kristin Scott Thomas, Hayden Christiansen). See previous section on adolescent individuation/rebellion' for movie description.

a   (1:37:41–1:41:54). George tells Sam that he has cancer. Sam feels that he has been 'tricked' by his father into spending this time together, not knowing until now what triggered his father's idea for them to build a house together.

b   (1:50:24–1:52:30). Sam visits his dying father in the hospital. With the help of an elaborate lighting system, he is able to show his father the progress on the house from his hospital bed.

1   What concerns would you have about a child or teen who is facing a parent's death?
2   Do you routinely arrange to see family members of a patient with a life-threatening illness? Why or why not?
3   What is your practice regarding contact with family members following the death of a patient?
4   What community resources are available to assist families?

# Chapter 4

# Adult developmental issues through the life cycle

*Patricia Lenahan*

Family physicians often encounter adult patients who experience distress related to life-cycle issues such as dating, marriage, pregnancy, child-rearing, launching children and facing losses. It is important for physicians to understand the significance of life-stage development for adults and families, and to recognize the interdependence of individuals within the family system.[1–4]

## Dating

◆ *Sleepless in Seattle* (Tom Hanks, Meg Ryan, Bill Pullman, Rosie O'Donnell, Rob Reiner, Ross Malinger, Caroline Aaron). Architect Sam Baldwin (Tom Hanks) portrays a widowed father who moves to Seattle with his son Jonah (Ross Malinger), who contacts Dr Marcia Fieldstone (Caroline Aaron), a talk-show host, to discuss his father's loneliness.

a (0:38:11–0:44:03). Sam is talking to a co-worker about dating. His friend wants to set him up with a date and he tells Sam that things have changed since Sam last dated. Sam admits that he hasn't dated since 'Jimmy Carter in 1978.' His friend tells him that the new dating means that you become friends first, then have tests and eventually get to do 'it' with a condom. He adds that you now split the check. Sam says he could never do that. The scene ends with Sam making a date.

1  What 'rules' do you have about dating?
2  What are some of the family expectations, traditions and values you have learned with regard to dating?
3  How would you advise a young widow/widower who expresses a desire to start dating?

## Engagement

◆ *Sleepless in Seattle* (Tom Hanks, Meg Ryan, Bill Pullman, Rosie O'Donnell, Rob Reiner, Ross Malinger, Caroline Aaron). See previous section on dating for movie description.

a (0:05:30–0:10:55). Writer Annie Reed (Meg Ryan) and her fiancé Walter (Bill Pullman) arrive at Annie's parents' home on Christmas Eve. They announce their engagement. The entire family becomes involved in discussing wedding plans.

Later, Annie's mother shows Annie her grandmother's wedding dress and talks about how she met Annie's father.

1 What stressors are associated with engagement?
2 How best can engaged couples maintain their independence from intrusive in-laws?
3 What intergenerational family values regarding marriage may be transmitted to engaged couples?

## Pregnancy and family formation

◆ *Nine Months* (Hugh Grant, Julianne Moore, Joan Cusack, Tom Arnold, Robin Williams, Jeff Goldblum). Child psychologist Sam Fulton (Hugh Grant) is happy with his five-year relationship with Rebecca (Julianne Moore). However, Sam's staid world goes askew when Rebecca becomes pregnant.

a (0:09:20–0:11:46). Rebecca and Sam are en route to a weekend get-together with friends. Rebecca tells Sam that she is pregnant. Sam drives off the road. Rebecca says to Sam, 'I guess you don't want the baby.' Sam chides her about not using birth control.

1 What is the impact of unplanned pregnancy on relationships?
2 How would you counsel a couple in this situation?
3 What would you tell someone about the efficacy of birth control methods?

b (0:13:02–0:15:50). Sam's friend Sean (Jeff Goldblum) says that his girlfriend left him because she wanted a child. Sean says that his ex-girlfriend would have 'swallowed my youth,' and compares her to a praying mantis that devours its mate.

1 What are the developmental tasks for young adults?
2 What advice would you give to a couple facing an unplanned pregnancy?

c (0:21:25–0:22:30). Sean complains that his brother-in-law Marty (Tom Arnold) and his sister Gail (Joan Cusack) used to be interesting people, but now all they talk about is kids.

1 How can couples maintain an adult marital relationship in the face of child-rearing demands?
2 What recommendations would you give expectant couples in this regard?

d (0:24:00–0:26:20). Sam plans to tell Rebecca that he does not want a child, but Rebecca pre-empts him by saying that she knows they are not ready for a child, but she still wants to keep it. She promises Sam that she will not let the baby change them.

1 How realistic is Rebecca's promise that the pregnancy will not change their relationship?
2 What are the developmental tasks for expectant families?

e (0:36:30–0:38:40). Rebecca tells Sam that they will need to get rid of his sports car and get a family car. She adds that he will also have to get rid of his 16-year-old cat because of hygiene issues. Sam responds by saying 'You said the baby wouldn't change our lives.'

1  How realistic was Rebecca's promise that their relationship would not change?
2  What advice would you give to a couple regarding pets in a home with infants and young children?

f  (0:43:19–0:47:45). Rebecca and Sam are having breakfast. He comments on how much she is eating. Rebecca says that she feels much better now that she is in the second trimester, and she apologizes for not having had sex for two months. She hints that maybe they could 'fool around' tonight. They engage in foreplay and Rebecca feels the baby move for the first time. Now she does not want to have sex, fearing that it will hurt the baby.

1  What are the risks of engaging in sexual activity during pregnancy?
2  At what point during pregnancy would you advise a couple to discontinue sex?
3  How would you respond to a couple's concerns that intercourse might harm the fetus?

g  (0:51:30–0:57:40). Sam forgets Rebecca's appointment for an ultrasound scan and arrives at the physician's office too late. The doctor tells Sam that he is having a son, and suggests that pregnant women need a lot of support. He gives him the videotape of the ultrasound scan that Rebecca had forgotten. Sam goes home and watches the tape.

1  What effect does watching the videotape of the ultrasound scan have on Sam?
2  What expectations (cultural, familial, etc.) do couples have based on the gender of the unborn child?

h  (1:09:05–1:14:40). Rebecca experiences premature contractions at seven months and is kept in hospital overnight for observation. Sam apologizes for being selfish because he is afraid of losing his youth. He tells Rebecca that he is in love with his child and that he has been reading Brazelton and has gone to a Lamaze class on his own.

1  How would you assess Sam's adjustment to the prospect of becoming a parent?
2  What educational material would you recommend to new parents?

i  (1:21:35–1:31:10). This is a truly comical scene in which Dr Kosevich (Robin Williams) is simultaneously dealing with Rebecca and her friend Gail (Joan Cusack). Both women are in labor. Gail's husband, Marty, is convinced that he will finally have a son. He is videotaping both his wife's labor and Rebecca's. The scene ends with Marty accepting another daughter and Rebecca and Sam admiring their son. Sam states that 'we're a family.'

1  What constitutes a family?
2  What are the developmental tasks for new parents?
3  How do these developmental tasks for new parents differ from those for a couple who have other children?
4  What advice would you give to both sets of parents?

## Launching children

◆ *Father of the Bride* (Diane Keaton, Steve Martin, Martin Short). This is a remake of the Spencer Tracy classic.

a (0:02:10–0:04:29). George Banks (Steve Martin) is seen after his daughter's wedding reminiscing about her growing up and meeting the right guy, and his losing her. He has been told that he will look back on his daughter's wedding day with affection and nostalgia.

b (0:09:20–0:13:43). Annie (Kimberley Williams) returns from a semester in Europe to announce her engagement. Her father (Steve Martin) has a flashback to Annie as a little girl. He asks what happened to her desire to get a job and be her own person. He is chided by his wife Nina (Diane Keaton), who tells him to stop acting like a lunatic father.

1  How would you characterize George's response to his daughter's engagement?
2  What are the developmental tasks for adolescents/young adults?

c (0:17:08–0:22:50). The Banks meet their future son-in-law, Brian McKenzie (George Newbern). While Nina succumbs to her daughter's happiness, George remains skeptical and reacts strongly when he observes Brian caressing his daughter's knee.

d (0:26:25–0:30:35). George and Nina meet Brian's parents for brunch. Brian's father says that it is hard to let your kids go and that you can only hope that you raised them right.

1  What is the role of parents in launching children?

e (0:36:00–0:40:04). Annie is discussing wedding plans with her parents and says that she wants to have the reception at home. George visualizes a barbecue wedding. Nina tells him that he has been acting crazy since their daughter announced her engagement, and she reminds him that a wedding is a 'big deal.'

f (1:15:30–1:19:53). It is the night before the wedding, and Annie's younger brother Mattie (Kieran Culkin) says to his father that it is 'just you, me and Mom here now.' The scene shifts to George in bed, seeing Annie from infancy through to announcing her engagement. George gets up and finds that Annie can't sleep either. She says that it is her last night in her house and her last night as a kid. She ends by saying 'I know I can't stay, but I don't want to go.'

g (1:27:45–1:28:38). George is walking his daughter down the aisle at the church. As he sits down, he realizes that Annie is leaving and that she is now grown up.

1  How do you understand George's ambivalence with regard to his daughter's wedding? How do you understand Annie's ambivalence?
2  What are some family expectations for weddings?
3  What traditions does your family have with regard to special occasions?
4  What variations in terms of wedding preparations and ceremony might you see based on an individual's cultural, ethnic or religious identity?

## Separation, divorce and remarriage

◆ *The Four Seasons* (Alan Alda, Carol Burnett, Sandy Dennis, Len Cariou, Rita Moreno, Jack Weston). This is the story of three middle-aged couples who are adjusting to the transitions in their lives.

a (0:16:20–0:20:40). The three couples are spending a weekend together to celebrate the twenty-first wedding anniversary of Nick (Len Cariou) and Annie (Sandy Dennis). In this scene Nick tells Jack (Alan Alda) that he should not have married Annie, and that it was painful to want to love someone for 20 years and not be able to do so. Nick says that the marriage is over and that he wants a new life, a new start, a new family and someone he can love. Jack asks how he thinks leaving his wife would affect Nick's daughter, Lisa. Nick says that she is 18 years old and she will understand.

1   What are the developmental tasks for middle-aged couples?
2   What impact does the 'empty-nest' syndrome have on couples?
3   What factors may lead to marital discord in couples who have been married for several years?

b (0:43:55–0:46:00). Nick gives his new girlfriend, Ginny (Bess Armstrong), a ring. This leads to a discussion between the other couples about relationships in middle age.

1   What are the expectations of couples during the middle years?
2   How would you respond to a couple who tell you that they want to feel happier in their relationship?
3   What is the impact of monotony on marital relationships?

c (0:50:56–0:53:00). The three couples are at a parents' weekend where Jack's daughter Beth (Elizabeth Alda) and Nick's daughter Lisa (Beatrice Alda) both attend college. Lisa meets her dad's new wife, Ginny. Jack comments that Lisa looks depressed. Nick responds that she is a survivor.

1   What is the impact of divorce and remarriage on children?
2   What are the development tasks for adolescence, and how are these impacted by a parental divorce?

d (1:03:00–1:06:06). Nick talks to his daughter Lisa about the divorce and remarriage. He acknowledges that he was affected by his parents' divorce and vowed that it would not happen to him. Lisa asks how he could make a decision that would affect her life. Nick gets upset and accuses her of 'emotional blackmail.'

1   What is the likelihood of family patterns repeating themselves?
2   In what way did Nick's divorce and remarriage affect his daughter?
3   What anticipatory guidance could you offer a couple contemplating divorce?

# Widowhood

◆ *Sleepless in Seattle* (Tom Hanks, Meg Ryan, Bill Pullman, Rosie O'Donnell, Rob Reiner, Ross Malinger). See earlier section on dating for movie description.

a (0:00:38–0:02:57). These opening scenes of the movie pan from images in the cemetery to family and friends consoling the newly widowed Sam (Tom Hanks). When his boss hands him a card for a therapist, Sam reacts emotionally and, referring to himself in the third person, says 'Don't mind him, he's just a guy who lost his wife.' Sam says that he needs a change of venue because everywhere he goes he sees his wife.

1 What is the impact of loss at this stage of the family life cycle?
2 How would you counsel a patient who has experienced loss at this age?
3 How would you address the issues of loss for children in the family?

b (0:13:01–0:17:43). Annie (Meg Ryan) is driving and listening to a talk radio station when Jonah (Ross Malinger) calls in and tells the host that his dad needs a new wife. Sam gets on the phone and explains that he and Jonah have had a rough time since his wife died. The talk-show therapist asks Sam how he is sleeping. Sam responds by telling her that it is Christmas, a time when his wife made everything special.

1 What are the stages of grief?
2 How can you distinguish between 'normal' bereavement and complicated bereavement?
3 What are the effects of holidays and special occasions on the grief response?
4 How would you provide anticipatory guidance to a widow/widower regarding reactions to holidays and special events?

c (0:28:16–0:29:06). It is New Year's Eve and Sam has put Jonah to bed. He lies on the couch and fantasizes about talking with his wife. He says that he misses her so much that it hurts.

1 How would you characterize Sam's reaction?
2 How would you respond to a patient who shared this experience with you?

## References

1. Sahler OJ, Carr JE, eds. *The Behavioral Sciences and Health Care.* Cambridge, MA: Hogrefe & Huber, 2003.
2. Sloane PD, Slatt LM, Ebell MH, Jacques LB. *Essentials of Family Medicine* (4e). Baltimore, MD: Lippincott Williams & Wilkins, 2002.
3. McDaniel S, Campbell TL, Lorenz A, Hepworth J. *Family-Oriented Primary Care* (2e). New York: Springer-Verlag, 2004.
4. Ratcliffe SD, Baxley EG, Byrd JE, Sakornbut EL, eds. *Family Practice Obstetrics* (2e). Philadelphia, PA: Hanley & Belfus, Inc, 2001.

# Chapter 5

# Family dynamics

*Matthew Alexander, Dael Waxman and Kathryn Fraser*

For a variety of reasons, understanding family dynamics is very important in the provision of healthcare.[1] Physical as well as mental problems tend to run in families. Family members provide important social and financial resources for individuals suffering from illness.[2] Conversely, family pathology often plays a role in the development and maintenance of illness.[2] Families hold and transmit to their youngest members certain key health beliefs that influence perception of illness as well as utilization of care.[3] Similarly, families practice and inculcate lifestyle behaviors that help (or hinder) compliance with health promotion.[3] Finally, individuals often turn to family experts for health advice, which may be at odds with that given by the healthcare provider.

For all of these reasons, it is critical that healthcare providers be educated about the impact of the family on healthcare. Relevant topics in this regard include:

- normal family functioning and dysfunctional families
- the individual life cycle and the family life cycle
- cross-cultural and changing demographic variations in the structure of the family
- skill in being 'family focused' when working with individuals
- knowing when and how best to involve family members in a patient's healthcare so as to improve outcomes.

Recent research has suggested that physicians with a family-oriented interviewing style (i.e. those who take time to learn about their patients' family and social contexts) are viewed by their patients as being knowledgeable about their history, health needs and values. This same research also found that physicians with a family-oriented style were more time efficient (i.e. spent less time with patients) than physicians with a family *history* style who focus on individuals and their medical histories rather than on family context.[4]

Cinemeducation has been linked with the education of healthcare professionals in family care.[5–8] This chapter strives to build on this previous work. The cinematic clips suggested below should be paired with appropriate readings in family systems concepts for maximal benefit.

## Family systems concepts

◆ *What's Eating Gilbert Grape?* (Johnny Depp, Leonardo DiCaprio, Mary Steenburgen, Juliette Lewis). This movie tells the story of the Grape family who live in the small rural community of Endora. This single-parent household consists of a morbidly obese mother (Darlene Cates), her mentally impaired son Arnie (Leonardo DiCaprio), his caretaking brother Gilbert (Johnny Depp), and their two sisters, Amy and Ellen. Juliette Lewis plays the out-of-town visitor who changes Gilbert's life.

a (0:01:30–0:06:13). In this scene we are introduced to the Grape family by Gilbert. He and his younger, mentally impaired brother, Arnie, are on the side of the road waiting for a caravan of campers to drive by. As the scene unfolds, Gilbert tells us about the town in which he lives and introduces us to the Grape family.

1 Draw a genogram of this nuclear family.
2 Draw a family circle from several family members' perspective.
3 At what stage is the Grape family in the family life cycle? By conventional standards, at what stage *should* they be? Are there cultural differences in the family life cycle? If so, what are they?
4 Describe the family 'homeostasis' in the Grape family, including important family alliances.
5 Give examples of parentification, enmeshment and geographical 'cut-offs' in this family.
6 What roles do the Grape family members play and how do these roles relate to each other?
7 Assume that Gilbert's mother is your patient. How do her symptoms influence the other family members?
8 How do the other family members influence the mother's symptoms?
9 As a family-oriented healthcare professional, how would you incorporate the family into the mother's ongoing treatment? What are the barriers to *change* in this family?

◆ *Ordinary People* (Donald Sutherland, Mary Tyler Moore, Judd Hirsch, Timothy Hutton). This is an award-winning movie about the impact of a son's death on an upper-middle-class family. The film tells the story of Beth (Mary Tyler Moore), an aloof mother and wife, Calvin (Donald Sutherland), a caring father, and Conrad (Timothy Hutton), their troubled teenage son who survives a tragic boating accident in which his brother is killed.

a (0:55:05–0:58:35). In this scene, Beth is at her parents' house with Calvin and Conrad. They are attempting to take family photographs, but Beth is very uncomfortable posing next to Conrad. After Conrad has an emotional 'melt-down,' Beth talks privately with her mother about him. Beth seems unable to have maternal feelings for Conrad or to reorganize her conception of her family without her oldest son.

1 How does this clip illustrate the concept of flexibility vs. rigidity in a family system?
2 How does this clip illustrate the concept of adaptability vs. resistance to change in a family system?
3 How does this clip illustrate the concept of an open vs. closed family system?
4 How does this clip illustrate emotional shut-down on the part of all family members?

◆ *The Great Santini* (Robert Duvall, Blythe Danner, Michael O'Keefe). This is a riveting film about Bull Meechum (Robert Duvall), a tough, ace Marine fighter pilot, his wife, Lillian (Blythe Danner), and their four children.

a (0:31:03–0:34:59). In this scene, Bull Meechum is unable to let his eldest son Ben (Michael O'Keefe) win a one-on-one basketball game with him.

1   What does this clip illustrate about coalitions within families?
2   What roles do Bull and Ben play in their family? What makes it so difficult for Bull to allow himself to lose this match? What does this scene illustrate about flexibility vs. rigidity in families as they proceed through the life cycle?
3   Is the father emotionally abusive (e.g. when he follows his son up the stairs and says 'You're my sweetest little girl')? How might you address such emotional abuse if you witnessed it in your office?

## Destructive interaction patterns/the alcoholic couple

◆   *Who's Afraid of Virginia Woolf?* (Richard Burton, Elizabeth Taylor). This movie is about a middle-aged alcoholic couple who have been married for many years. They have a highly conflictual and antagonistic relationship. The intensity of their negative interactions is heightened by their abuse of alcohol.

a (0:34:36–0:40:03). Martha (Elizabeth Taylor) and George (Richard Burton) invite a young couple over for drinks after an evening out, and then proceed to humiliate each other by dredging up hurtful things they have done to each other in the past. They show extremely poor judgement, and thus poor boundaries, by airing their 'dirty laundry' in front of people they barely know. In this scene, George takes out what people initially believe is a gun and aims it at Martha. It opens up into an umbrella and then everyone laughs. This scene is quite extreme and offers some of the best 'couples trashing' ever captured on film.

1   What is your reaction to this couple? What should be the first step towards helping them?
2   How does this scene illustrate the concept of runaway escalation (i.e. rapidly increasing patterns of negative interaction)? What is the best advice to give couples and families who frequently experience such emotional escalations in their homes?
3   What impact does alcohol have on domestic disputes?
4   What does this couple's behavior demonstrate about their ability to communicate with each other? Are there different norms in different families with regard to acceptable public behavior?

## Boundaries

◆   *About Schmidt* (Jack Nicholson, Kathy Bates). Warren Schmidt (Jack Nicholson) plays a newly retired husband and father whose life undergoes a dramatic change when his wife dies suddenly. Upon his wife's death, Schmidt becomes fixated on the need to abort his adult daughter's imminent wedding to an underachieving waterbed salesman.

a (1:16:55–1:22:25). In this scene, Schmidt meets the groom's eccentric mother (Kathy Bates) for the second time. She has an 'off-camera' fight with Larry, her ex-husband, and subsequently reveals more personal information to Schmidt than he (or anyone else for that matter) would care to know.

b (1:34:40–1:37:04). The groom's mother is feeding Schmidt after he has sprained his neck. She reveals detailed personal information about her own sex life and that of Schmidt's daughter and soon-to-be son-in-law.

1 In what way are these scenes examples of poor boundaries? What are other examples of poor/crossed boundaries within families?
2 Why is the issue of boundaries such an important one within families?
3 How can healthcare professionals tell when a patient has poor boundaries in relation to them?
4 How can healthcare professionals establish good boundaries with their patients?

◆ *Ordinary People* (Mary Tyler Moore, Donald Sutherland, Judd Hirsch, Timothy Hutton). See previous section on family systems concepts for movie description.

a (0:31:12–0:32:42). Calvin and Beth are attending a party together. Calvin reveals to a friend that Conrad is seeing a therapist. Beth overhears and joins them to change the subject of the conversation. During the ride home, Beth is angry and feels that Calvin violated the family's privacy.

1 What are the 'proper' boundaries concerning public discussion of personal family matters?
2 How well does this couple resolve their disagreement? What suggestions would you make for their coming to a better future understanding about how to handle family information that one spouse considers to be private?
3 What are other areas of family history and functioning that families often keep hidden from others?
4 What impact do family secrets (i.e. personal family matters that are considered shameful and are therefore hidden from others) have on family members?

## Family breakdown

◆ *The Story of Us* (Michelle Pfeiffer, Bruce Willis). This movie tells the story of Ben (Bruce Willis) and Katie (Michelle Pfeiffer), the married parents of two children, and their struggles in deciding whether or not to stay married.

a (0:06:30–0:07:22). While out for an anniversary dinner with Ben, Katie reflects on the history of conflict in their marriage.

1 What role does fighting play in a committed relationship? How does one distinguish between 'fair' and destructive fighting? How do words such as 'always' and 'never' contribute to misunderstandings between couples?
2 What are some of the root causes of the fighting between *this* couple? As a healthcare provider, how would you help this couple to address their issues (i.e. *his* feelings that she never lets go of the past and *her* feelings that he never listens)?
3 What are some other common causes of fighting in committed relationships?
4 As a healthcare professional, would you ever counsel a couple to divorce? If so, when and how would you make such a suggestion?
5 If either of these individuals were your medical patient, when and how would you recommend marital counseling? To whom would you send them?

6 As a healthcare professional, in what ways can you help couples to avoid marital breakdown?

◆ *Who's Afraid of Virginia Woolf* (Elizabeth Taylor, Richard Burton). See previous section on destructive interaction patterns/the alcoholic couple for movie description.

a (0:13:23–0:15:05). In this scene, George and Martha are drinking and being playful in bed. George rejects Martha's attempt at physical intimacy.

1 How does this scene illustrate the negative impact of unresolved conflict, criticism and contempt on couples? What is the best advice for couples whose disagreements escalate out of control?
2 How do unresolved sexual issues impact marital harmony?
3 What are the optimal ways for couples to resolve issues related to differences in intimacy needs?
4 What are some reasons for low sexual desire in committed couples? Is low sexual desire more common in men or in women? How is this problem best treated?
5 What advice can you give to couples who present with mismatches in sexual desire?
6 Is there a medical problem that George may be avoiding by refusing Martha's advances?

## Intergenerational patterns

◆ *The Story of Us* (Michelle Pfeiffer, Bruce Willis). See previous section on family breakdown for movie description.

a (0:37:54–0:40:45). Ben and Katie are trying to be intimate after a separation.

Side by side on their bed, they reminisce about a psychoanalyst who once informed them that there are always 'six' people (i.e. the couple plus their respective sets of parents) in a couple's bedroom. The scene progresses to show Ben and Katie resurfacing old issues with each other. As their fight escalates, the viewer sees each set of parents weighing in. We suggest that the clip be viewed twice in succession.

### First viewing

1 How are Ben and Katie similar to their respective parents?
2 What impact does our family of *origin* have on our family of *creation*? How is this impact illustrated in this scene?
3 How can couples avoid repeating intergenerational patterns in their relationship?
4 When might a physician find it helpful to enquire about a patient's family of origin?

## Second viewing

1 How do Ben and Katie move from joking to screaming in a matter of minutes?
2 What is the best advice for couples who escalate their arguments so rapidly?
3 How could this argument have been avoided?
4 How can couples learn from past mistakes without repeating them?
5 Have you ever lost your temper with a patient? What happened? How did it feel afterwards?

# Impact of chronic illness on family

◆ *Safe* (Julianne Moore). This movie tells the story of Carol White (Julianne Moore), a suburban housewife with a mysterious chronic illness.

a (0:28:28–0:30:33). In this scene, Carol and her husband are getting ready for bed. She declines his invitation to have sexual relations as she does not feel well.

1 What is the impact of Carol's illness on the relationship?
2 Do you think Carol's clinician knows how her illness is affecting the family?
3 How would you ask about the impact of an illness on a patient's family?
4 What is the possible *function* of the illness in the family context?

◆ *Steel Magnolias* (Sally Field, Dolly Parton, Shirley MacLaine, Julia Roberts). This movie, set in a Southern town, is the story of Shelby (Julia Roberts), a dynamic woman with diabetes, and her mother, M'lynn (Sally Field). M'lynn worries about the impact that the stress-filled wedding planning may have on Shelby's health.

a (0:17:40–0:28:19). In this scene, Shelby and her mother are having their hair done at the local hair salon in preparation for Shelby's wedding. Together all of the women discuss the wedding details. Shelby and M'Lynn disagree about almost everything. Shelby becomes weak and experiences hypoglycemia.

1 How does this scene illustrate the family systems concepts of over- and under-functioning?
2 Is M'Lynn enmeshed with her daughter? If so, why? Does chronic illness in a child make this a more likely outcome? Why? How can enmeshment in such circumstances be avoided or minimized?
3 If Shelby was your patient and her mother was accompanying her on a visit to you, how would you avoid becoming triangulated by them?
4 How would you take a family-focused approach to assist Shelby in becoming more compliant with her medical regimen?
5 How does this scene illustrate aspects of the *functional* as opposed to *structural* family? How can one learn more about a patient's functional family?

# Balancing roles

◆ *Ordinary People* (Mary Tyler Moore, Donald Sutherland, Judd Hirsch, Timothy Hutton). See previous section on family systems concepts for movie description.

a (0:23:56–0:25:01). In this scene, Beth and Calvin try to decide whether or not to spend their Christmas vacation in London. Calvin expresses doubt about this being a good time to go away, particularly since their son, Conrad, would miss three weeks of therapy. Beth feels that keeping the family tradition is important.

1  Suppose that this couple asked you for your professional opinion to settle their dilemma. What advice would you offer?
2  What personal feelings do you notice having towards each parent's viewpoint? Could there be positive benefits from the family getting away after the trauma that they have incurred?
3  Could going away now also be seen as a way to sabotage/devalue treatment? Do you think that their son's opinion should be solicited? Why or why not?
4  How would you counsel couples to balance their roles as *parents* with their roles as *spouses*?
5  What are the advantages and disadvantages of a 'marriage-focused' family? What are the advantages and disadvantages of a 'child-focused' family? Is one approach better than the other?

## References

1. Sawa R. *Family Health Care*. Newbury Park, CA: Sage Publications, 1992.
2. National Institute of Mental Health. Series DN No. 6. Families Impact on Health: a critical review and annotated bibliography by TL Campbell. DNSS Pub. No. (ADM) 86-1461. Washington DC: Supt. of Docs., US Govt. Print off, 1986.
3. Doherty WJ, Baird MA. *Family Therapy and Family Medicine*. New York: Guilford Press, 1983.
4. Gotler RS, Medalie JH, Zyzanski SJ *et al.* Focus on the family. Part 2: Does a family focus affect patient outcomes? *Fam Pract Manage* 2001; **8**: 45–6.
5. Alexander M, Waxman D. Cinemeducation: teaching family systems through the movies. *Fam Systems Health* 2000; **18**: 455–62.
6. Bayard P. Teaching family therapy theory: do something different. *Am J Fam Ther* 1996; **24**: 195–205.
7. Higins JA, Dermer S. The use of film in marriage and family counselor education. *Counsel Educ Supervis* 2001; **40**: 182–92.
8. Hudock AM, Warden SA. Using movies to teach family systems concepts. *Fam J Counsel Ther Couples Fam* 2001; **9**: 116–21.

# Chapter 6

# A life cycle approach to sexuality

*Amy Ellwood, Patricia Lenahan and Anna Pavlov*

Sexuality is an integral aspect of life. Intimacy, sensuality and sexual expression begin during the earliest stages of development and continue until the end of life. Sexuality and what is viewed as 'normal' sexual expression vary a great deal from person to person. Sexual desire itself is mediated by differences in the sex drive, and may be affected by interpersonal, intrapersonal, cultural and religious influences.

Family physicians serve a vital role in providing knowledge, understanding and education about sexuality to their patients as they progress through the life cycle. Parents of young children may need assistance in understanding masturbatory behaviors in their children. Adolescents may engage in sexual behavior as a way of demonstrating their independence, yet they often lack the maturity, knowledge or sense of responsibility necessary for mature sexuality. In both adolescents *and* adults, unplanned pregnancies and sexually transmitted diseases (e.g. herpes, HIV) may result from engaging in unprotected sexual intercourse. Pregnancy itself may cause couples to change their sexual patterns and behaviors. Pregnant couples look to their physicians to provide them with *information* about sex and *permission* to engage in sexual behavior during this time. Finally, individuals frequently experience the onset of chronic illness during the fifth and sixth decades of life. They may experience sexual difficulties as a result of either physical changes in health status or psychological issues related to their illness. Family physicians can serve a vital role in normalizing these difficulties and helping patients to find ways to manage them successfully.

This chapter focuses on common life cycle sexual issues in heterosexuals (*see* Chapter 23 for a discussion of issues relevant to GLBT (gay, lesbian, bisexual, transgender individuals). Trigger questions in both chapters might apply to all groups. Please note that the video clips may contain sexual language, nudity or individuals/couples engaged in sexual acts. It is important to inform the audience about this prior to showing these scenes.

## Adolescent sexuality

### Gender differences

◆ *Kids* (Leo Fitzpatrick, Justin Pierce, Chloe Sevigny, Rosario Dawson). This is a very powerful and disturbing film that looks at a day in the lives of several urban teenagers who are experimenting with drugs and sex. It provides a vivid insight into the thought processes of teenagers, their feelings of invincibility and the fallacy of their cognitions. This film is raw and real – it is not a film for the faint-hearted.

a (0:13:30–0:15:50, 0:16:50–0:18:00, 0:18:46–0:19:44). In these clips we see a group of girls talking about their first sexual experiences, what they want compared with what the boys want, and the types of sex in which they have engaged.

1  What is your emotional reaction to this scene?
2  How do your personal feelings about adolescent sexuality affect the physician–patient relationship?
3  How would you counsel adolescents about safer sex?
4  Were you surprised by the age of the girls and the range of their sexual activities?

b (0:15:50–0:16:46, 0:18:05–0:18:45). In these clips the boys share their sexual encounters and complain that girls want you to be 'caring and kind.'

1  What kind of reaction does this scene evoke in you?
2  What differences do you see in the behaviors, experiences and expectations of boys and girls, based on their conversations?

## Condom use

a (0:19:48–0:21:10). The discussion turns to condoms and how they don't work. The group feels that condoms are unnecessary because they don't know anyone who has died of AIDS.

1  How would you counsel an adolescent about condom use?
2  What strategies could you employ to encourage teenagers to address the risks of unprotected sex?

## Invincibility

a (0:21:15–0:22:25, 0:25:03–0:26:21). These clips follow two girls who are going to be tested for sexually transmitted diseases (STDs). Jenny (Chloe Sevigny) accompanies her friend Ruby (Rosario Dawson) as a gesture of support, and decides to get tested as well. She is not worried because she has only had sex with one boy while her friend has had multiple partners. When they return to the clinic for the test results, Ruby is told that she has no STDs. However, Jenny is told that she is HIV-positive.

1  What factors are associated with the early onset of sexuality among adolescents?
2  How can family physicians promote discussions of health and sexuality in their practice?
3  Forming a sexual identity is a key developmental task of adolescence. What educational strategies can the family physician employ in educating both parents and adolescents about the formation of sexual identity?
4  Since invincibility is characteristic of adolescence, how can you encourage sexually active teenagers to use condoms or be abstinent?
5  How well did the healthcare worker break the news to Jenny that she was HIV-positive? What types of counseling need to be offered when informing a patient that he or she is HIV-positive?

## Masturbation

◆ *Raising Victor Vargas* (Victor Rasuk, Judy Marte, Melonie Diaz, AltaGracia Guzman, Silvestre Rasuk). In this 'coming-of-age' film, Victor is an 18-year-old who lives in a one-bedroom apartment with his grandmother, brother and half-sister. His mother is a drug addict and his father is deceased. His grandmother, who emigrated to New York from the Dominican Republic, is the legal guardian. She does not trust Victor, and she suspects that he is a bad influence on his younger brother, Nino, who worships him.

a (0:27:15–0:29:38). Nino asks Victor for advice about girls. Victor comments on his brother's chapped lips and advises him that girls look at lips. Nino then asks Victor about masturbation. Their conversation is interrupted when their grandmother walks into the room.

b (0:48:00–0:48:55). The grandmother walks in on her younger grandson masturbating in the bathroom. He says that he is only using the bathroom, but she saw him and proceeds to say she is 'so ashamed.' She then scolds him and asks if that is what his brother has been teaching him.

c (1:09:38–1:12:12). Victor has his girlfriend, Judy, over for a family dinner. His grandmother becomes upset when she realizes that Judy has been to their apartment before without her knowledge. She accuses Victor of putting ideas into his younger sister's head about boys (rushing her development) and causing Nino to masturbate ('I caught my baby in the bathroom') and threatens to change the lock on the door.

1 How would you respond to a teenager who trusted you enough to ask whether it was normal to masturbate?
2 How would you respond to a parent or grandparent who reacted similarly to Victor's grandmother?
3 What suggestions might you make to a parental figure who believes that self-stimulation is immoral and violates religious principles (as does Victor's grandmother)?

## Infertility

◆ *Hannah and Her Sisters* (Woody Allen, Mia Farrow). This film provides a window into the lives of Hannah (Mia Farrow) and her sisters while they cope with their chemically dependent family of origin. One of the issues facing Hannah is her husband's infertility and their inability to conceive. Her husband, Mickey (Woody Allen), is a hypochondriac, and his infertility adds yet another insult to his already low self-esteem.

a (0:32:30–0:36:24). The couple receives the bad news that Mickey has an inadequate sperm count. He blames himself and speculates that his masturbating caused the low sperm count. Mickey and Hannah ask a married friend if he will agree to be a sperm donor for them.

1 What are people's common beliefs about infertility? What is the impact of infertility on self-esteem?

2 What are the different ways in which various cultural groups might perceive and experience this 'problem'?

3 What is the long-term impact of infertility on the marital and sexual functioning of couples?

## Erectile dysfunction

Erectile dysfunction has become medicalized. Relationship issues and the shame and embarrassment of seeking help for this problem are rarely discussed in exchange for the 'little blue pill.' In fact, psychosocial issues always need to be considered when evaluating and treating erectile dysfunction.

◆ *Same Time Next Year* (Alan Alda, Ellen Burstyn). This movie focuses on the long-term affair of George (Alan Alda) and Doris (Ellen Burstyn), who meet once a year for an extramarital romance that continues over the course of their lifetime.

a (0:52:30–0:55:00). George discloses to Doris that his wife Helen 'broke his pecker' and he is unable to become aroused.

1 What are some psychological reasons for erectile dysfunction?

2 What are the variety of treatment approaches available for men who are experiencing erectile dysfunction?

## Sex in pregnancy

◆ *Same Time Next Year*. See previous section on erectile dysfunction for movie description.

a. (0:48:00–0:51:00). George is eagerly awaiting their sexual reunion. Doris arrives and reveals that she is eight months pregnant. They discuss the sexual creativity they will need for this reunion because of her pregnancy.

b (0:55:30–0:59:30). Doris is physically uncomfortable being eight months pregnant, and George is rubbing her feet as they talk. He becomes sexually aroused, jumps up and moves across the room with anxiety. He wonders if he is perverted because a 200-pound pregnant woman sexually arouses him.

1 What beliefs do people have about hurting a pregnant woman or her fetus during sexual encounters?

2 Are there any particular sexual acts that should be avoided during pregnancy?

## Anorgasmia

◆ *Bliss* (Craig Shiffer, Sheryl Lee, Terence Stamp, Spalding Gray). This movie focuses on the relationship between Maria (Sheryl Lee) and her husband, Joseph (Craig Shiffer). Joseph accepts that Maria engages in some obsessive-compulsive behaviors, 'gets suicidal from time to time' and sleeps with a fly swatter. However, when she tells him that she is faking orgasms, the couple is sent down a road of self-discovery.

**a** (0:05:00–0:07:45). Maria and Joseph are in a therapy session and Maria complains that Joseph is not nice to either her family or her friends. Then, when Maria states that she wants to have a baby, Alfred (Spalding Gray), the therapist, asks about the quality of their sexual relationship. Maria confesses to Joseph that she has never had an orgasm with him. While they are lying in bed, Joseph asks Maria if she thinks that he is a lousy lover.

**b** (0:13:35–0:16:17). Maria tells Joseph that she still enjoys making love with him even if she cannot have an orgasm. The scene shifts to a therapy session where Joseph complains about Maria's numerous telephone calls to him at work. Maria leaves the session after stating that she cannot handle it when he gets so angry. The therapist then asks Joseph what he wants. Later, it is revealed that Maria's problems stem from her having been molested by her father.

1   What aspects of a sexual history are important to obtain when working with a patient like Maria?
2   What physician behaviors allow patients to feel safe to address sexual concerns?
3   What are the various causes of non-orgasmia in women? What are the appropriate treatments?
4   What are the long-term sexual consequences of childhood sexual abuse?
5   What is the role of the family physician in identifying and treating victims of childhood sexual abuse?

## Sexuality and breast cancer

◆ *A Thousand Acres* (Jason Robards, Jessica Lange, Michelle Pfieffer, Jennifer Jason Leigh). Based on the book with the same title, *A Thousand Acres* has been compared to a modern-day King Lear. Larry Cook (Jason Robards), a farmer and aging widower, decides to divide his farm among his three daughters. As the story unfolds, family history and dysfunction are revealed as Larry reels at the perceived rejection of his daughters.

a   (0:16:10–0:18:06). Rose (Michelle Pfeiffer), who has had a mastectomy, is receiving her one-month check-up with the oncologist. As he is checking her strength, she tells him that she still feels lopsided. She is clearly worried, and implies that her husband is not interested in her sexually. The physician focuses on her physical health and does not respond to her psychosocial or sexual concerns. In the scene following this clip, it is revealed that Rose's mother died of breast cancer.

1   What is the role of the primary care physician in counseling women about psychosexual issues following a mastectomy?
2   What is the impact of breast cancer on sexual functioning?
3   How does chemotherapy affect sexual functioning and desire?
4   The patient's spouse may be having difficulty coping with his wife's illness. What types of psychoeducational resources or therapies would you suggest for partners and family members of breast cancer patients?
5   Would your approach to this patient be different if she was unpartnered or lesbian?

# Sex and disability

◆ *Coming Home* (Bruce Dern, Jane Fonda, John Voigt). Marine Captain Bob Hyde (Bruce Dern) is sent to Vietnam, leaving his wife Sally (Jane Fonda) to fend for herself. Sally is encouraged to volunteer at the local base hospital, where she meets Luke Martin (John Voigt), a former sergeant. He is angry and frustrated because of a war injury that has left him a paraplegic. Over time, Luke and Sally develop a relationship that continues to grow in intimacy.

a (1:24:00–1:27:25). In this clip, the relationship between Sally and Luke has reached the point of physical intimacy. The scene opens with Luke going into the bathroom to prepare for their sexual encounter. Luke directs Sally to place the sheepskin mat on the bed. Sally asks where she can touch him and what he can feel.

1   How important is communication in achieving a satisfying level of sexual intimacy?
2   What are some of the common perceptions regarding the sexuality and sensuality of individuals with physical limitations?
3   What is the role of fantasy in sexual encounters?

◆ *The Waterdance* (Eric Stoltz, Helen Hunt, Wesley Snipes). Joel Garcia (Eric Stoltz) awakens in hospital following a hiking accident that has left him paralyzed. He has been placed on a physical medicine and rehabilitation unit where he will be taught how to adjust to his new life.

a (0:28:17–0:29:35). A spinal-cord-injured physician gives a sex talk to the patients and their partners. He discusses the effects of spinal cord injury on sexual function and mentions reflex erections. When the doctor states that 'oral sex comes in handy' there are myriad reactions from the patients. Raymond (Wesley Snipes), in particular, states that 'brothers don't do that.'

1   What cultural or religious factors may affect a patient's ability to consider alternative forms of sexual activity/satisfaction?
2   What is the role of the physician in discussing sexuality with patients who have chronic illnesses or injuries that may affect their sexual functioning?
3   What is the role of the partner?

b (0:40:04–0:43:57). Joel and Anna (Helen Hunt), his married girlfriend, are playing Scrabble. She begins to caress his arm, which leads to heavy petting and they close the curtain between them and the other patients in the ward. As their lovemaking progresses, other patients begin to hear their sighs. A nurse stands outside the curtain and says 'Knock, knock . . . medication time. I hope I'm not interrupting anything.'

c (0:45:21–0:46:10). The nurse stops Anna as she is leaving and says 'We understand the patient's need for sex therapy, but on the ward . . .'. She seems somewhat uncomfortable, and continues, 'there's something about insurance . . .'.

1   What accommodation can be made to provide privacy for patients and their partners in hospital settings?

2  What can the physician do to enhance quality-of-life issues for patients and their families?

**d** (0:51:05–0:53:16). Joel has a pass from the rehabilitation facility, and he immediately stops at the Tahiti Motel with Anna. He spends a lot of time looking at her before he begins touching her. She is somewhat uncomfortable and shy, but she acquiesces. As their lovemaking proceeds, the appliance for collecting urine slips off. Joel, embarrassed and angry, is too distraught to continue. Anna tries to soothe him, and tells him that they can start again, but Joel resists, stating that he cannot feel anything anyway.

1  What counseling strategies would you employ to help to prepare a couple for their first sexual encounter after a spinal cord injury?
2  What preparations do spinal-cord-injured patients need to make before sexual encounters? What equipment can be recommended to facilitate successful sexual encounters?
3  How would you involve the partner in educational sessions with regard to sexual adaptation to spinal cord injury?

◆  *The Theory of Flight* (Helena Bonham Carter, Kenneth Branagh). Richard (Kenneth Branagh), a disgruntled artist, is sentenced to 100 hours of community service, where he meets Jane (Helena Bonham Carter), a young woman with amyotrophic lateral sclerosis (ALS). Jane makes an unusual request. She wants Richard to help her to have sex before she loses all sensation and ability to perform.

**a** (0:10:12–0:11:05). The scene pans Jane's room at home, the hospital bed and her medications, etc. You hear sexual sounds coming from her computer and see Jane watching a sexually explicit film as her mother enters the room.

1  Why is pornography controversial? What are the various views regarding the use of pornography?
2  What role can watching sexually explicit movies serve in the lives of disabled individuals?
3  How would you respond to a patient who asks you what you think about viewing pornography or other sexually explicit films?

**b** (0:32:48–0:39:04). Using her electronic voice machine, Jane explains to Richard that she has not always been like this, and she asks him for a favor. Jane says her biggest regret is not having sex with her boyfriend when she was 17 years old. She says she knows that Richard is familiar with London, and she tells him that she knows 'There are places in London where people can have sex.' She asks Richard to help her lose her virginity. Richard is taken aback and wonders if Jane can have sexual relations. Jane replies that she cannot pleasure herself any more, but that her illness has not affected her sense of touch.

1  What would you say to a patient who expresses concern that they will never again be able to experience physical/genital sex?
2  How does a person's body image impact upon their sexual identity?
3  What recommendations would you make to patients whose disabilities interfere with their sexual functioning?

c (0:44:56–0:46:30). Jane is looking at an online dating service. The scene shows her typing 'Hideously crippled woman seeks sex . . .'.

1 How does a person's body image affect their feelings about life in general?
2 What cautions or advice would you give to a patient regarding online dating services?
3 How does Jane's self-concept affect other areas of her life?

d (0:47:14–0:50:12). Richard has agreed to help Jane to have sex. They visit a series of agencies and finally a club where a number of people are in wheelchairs. Jane becomes upset and wants to leave – she wants to be normal and have sex with a normal person. While discussing her fantasies as they approach their hotel, Jane sees a man (a gigolo) getting out of a limousine. She says that this is the person with whom she wants to have sex.

1 What personal values and feelings would influence your response to a patient who shares with you the fact that they have been with a prostitute?
2 What feelings does Jane's desperation for sex evoke in you?
3 How would you help Jane to cope with her desire to be normal?

# Sex and aging

## Menopause

◆ *Real Women Have Curves* (America Ferrera, Lupe Ontiveros, Ingrid Olin, Brian Sites). This movie is the story of an overweight Latina who struggles between her desire to go to college and her obligation to meet the family's expectations and needs.

a (1:07:00–1:08:10). Ana (America Ferrera) accompanies her mother, Carmen (Lupe Ontiveros), to the doctor's office. Carmen has been insisting that she is pregnant because she has not had a period for three months. The physician gently explains that it is not unusual for a woman of her age (51 years) to miss periods. He suggests that they talk about the menopause. Carmen reacts strongly and says that her life is over and she is no longer a woman.

1 What is the role of culture in understanding the experience of the menopause? How has our view of the menopause shifted to one of greater openness and acceptance (e.g. more books on the subject, support groups, etc.)?
2 What are some of the myths about the menopause?
3 What is the impact of the menopause on the sexual response cycle?
4 What factors contribute to decreased sexual activity in postmenopausal women?
5 What recommendations can you give postmenopausal women to enhance their sexual experiences?

## Sexual desire and activity in later life

Sexual desire and activity continue well into later life for both men and women, yet many physicians ignore this important part of life in their geriatric patients.

◆ *Grumpy Old Men* (Jack Lemmon, Walter Matthau, Ann Margret, Burgess Meredith). This film is about the renewal of romance in two retired men, and their competition for the exciting and available woman who has moved into their neighborhood.

a (0:13:30–0:14:10). John Gustafson (Jack Lemmon) tells his father (Burgess Meredith) that he has a new neighbor, Ariel (Ann Margret). Mr Gustafson asks him if he has mounted her yet, and John is appalled at his father's brash comment.

b (0:43:00–0:44:08). John prepares for an evening of romance with Ariel, but Max (Walter Matthau) gets to Ariel's door first. It is the first time in decades that either John or Max has romanced a woman, and they are both excited about their prospects of finding romance.

c (1:02:00–1:04:51). Ariel visits John and invites him to go to bed. John experiences anxiety and wonders about 'safe sex.'

1 What is the most common reason for lack of sexual interaction in geriatric populations?
2 When prescribing medication for erectile dysfunction to a geriatric patient, what medical and psychological issues should be considered?
3 Should elderly people be concerned with safe-sex practices?

## Alternative sexual subcultures

◆ *The Secretary* (Maggie Gyllenhaal, James Spader). Lee Holloway (Maggie Gyllenhaal), a young woman with a history of self-mutilation (cutting) and dependency, takes a job as a secretary. Her boss, Edward Gray (James Spader), is reserved and aloof until he begins involving her in a sadomasochistic relationship.

a (0:47:50–0:52:45). Lee makes some errors in a report for Mr Gray. He tells her to bend over the desk and he then spanks her hard. Initially she seems shocked at his response to her mistakes, but she then begins to enjoy the spanking. Afterwards she goes to the bathroom to look at the red marks left on her buttocks.

b (0:56:41–0:58:10). Lee is at home reading *Cosmopolitan* magazine while pleasuring herself. She is fantasizing about a romantic relationship with Mr Gray that includes sadomasochism and submission.

c (1:27:50–1:28:30). Lee responds to ads for people interested in BDSM (bondage, discipline and sadomasochism). The scene shows several individuals talking about or engaged in BDSM and urophilic acts.

1 Is there a relationship between BDSM and dysfunctional behaviors such as cutting?
2 How would you counsel a patient who participates in alternative sexual subcultures?
3 What health-related concerns would you have for a patient who participates in alternative sexual subcultures?
4 How do your personal values and beliefs affect your approach to and treatment of a patient who engages in alternative sexual expression?

# Sexual addiction

◆ *Auto Focus* (Greg Kinnear, Willem DaFoe). This film is based on the life of Bob Crane (Greg Kinnear), the television star of *Hogan's Heroes*, and depicts his descent into sexual addiction. His association with a video technician, John Carpenter (Willem DaFoe), and his celebrity enable his addiction to advance. As Crane attempts to recover, he is brutally murdered.

a (0:31:00–0:32:05). John is showing Bob the videotape from their night with two women. Bob is admiring the taping system and becoming sexually aroused as he views himself receiving oral sex. He tells John that he wants a taping system.

1 What impact does Bob's relationship with John have on him?
2 What are the legal and ethical issues with regard to this situation?

b (0:35:16–0:36:26). Bob is being interviewed for a Christian publication. He is asked how he has managed to stay married for 15 years. We then see Bob having sex with multiple partners and narrating how he reduces stress through sex, a 'harmless safety valve.' Bob responds to the interviewer by saying that, when it comes to his family, he 'doesn't make waves.'

1 What role does denial play in sex addiction?
2 How would you respond to Bob's perception that his sexual behavior reduces stress and is 'harmless'?
3 As Bob's physician, what precautions would you recommend?
4 Would you have any ethical/legal obligation with regard to Bob's wife?

c (0:53:17–0:55:05). Bob returns home to be confronted by his wife, Anne. She is very upset and presents Bob with nude photos of different women, which she found in his dark room.

1 How does sex addiction affect the family? If Anne was your patient and told you what she had found, how would you respond to her?
2 How might the impact of sex addiction differ from that of other addictions such as alcoholism or drug abuse?
3 What resources are available to assist families with this problem?

d (1:06:53–1:08:06). John stops by to see Bob. They talk about making a pornographic film. Bob insists on showing John his enhanced penis. Their mantra becomes 'a day without sex is a day wasted.'

1 How would you assess a patient who has asked about obtaining a penile enhancement?
2 How might signs of sexual addiction surface in an office visit?
3 What might a partner of a sexually addicted patient complain of?

e (1:13:25–1:16:00). John drops in at Bob's house and finds him in the basement editing videos. Bob is wearing boxer shorts. He discloses to John that he and his wife are having problems. As they watch the video, Bob masturbates while he and John are talking and trying to remember what city they were in when the tape was made.

1 What is your reaction to this scene?
2 What does this scene communicate about the nature of sexual addiction?

Chapter 7

# Chronic illness

*Joseph Kertesz and Anna Pavlov*

The incidence of chronic disease is continuing to rise. Chronic illness exacts a considerable physical, social, emotional and financial toll on the individual and the family. Chronic disease can affect individuals at any time during the course of the family life cycle. As such, it can impact on the family's functioning in numerous and unexpected ways and challenge the family's adaptability and resilience.

As life expectancy increases, chronic disease becomes more commonplace as illness to be *managed* rather than cured. The management of chronic disease, by definition, implies longevity of the doctor–patient relationship. Family physicians have a unique opportunity to offer a supportive environment in which to assist patients and families who are dealing with the challenges imposed by chronic illness.[1]

Although several psychiatric conditions, such as depression and schizophrenia, are viewed as chronic illnesses, this chapter will focus on chronic medical conditions such as asthma, diabetes and stroke. Other disorders and conditions which are chronic in nature, such as Alzheimer's disease, are discussed elsewhere in this book.

## Pediatric chronic illness (asthma), parent and child issues

◆ *As Good as it Gets* (Jack Nicholson, Helen Hunt, Skeet Ulrich). This film depicts the unlikely relationship between an initially toxic and unlikable writer with obsessive-compulsive disorder, Melvin Udall (Jack Nicholson), and a no-nonsense waitress, Carol (Helen Hunt), who is a single parent of a child, Spencer (Skeet Ulrich), with chronic and severe asthma. Carol finds support for her son's care in the most unlikely of places. The film portrays the physical, emotional and financial struggles of parenting a child with a chronic illness.

a (0:21:30–0:22:55). Melvin is making his daily breakfast stop at the restaurant where Carol regularly waits on him. He asks what is wrong with her son. Carol explains how he 'has to fight to breathe . . . and how an ear infection sends us to the ER five or six times a month.'

1 What are the issues affecting a parent whose child has a chronic illness?
2 What can family physicians do to recognize/identify these issues and assist parents?
3 What community resources are available to assist the families of children with chronic illness?

b (0:33:05–0:33:58). Melvin enquires in an unflattering way about Carol's tired appearance. She explains that she has been up all night with her son, who had a 'full-blown attack' and received the wrong antibiotic.

1 How often do we discuss self-care issues with parents?
2 What can we do to assist parents/families in circumstances in which they have few resources?
3 What cultural, ethnic and religious values may impact on treatment and/or utilization of ancillary services?

c (0:51:50–0:55:50). Carol runs home to find a pediatric specialist and a private nurse attending her son. She is overcome with disbelief and joy at her good fortune, until she learns that Melvin is responsible for arranging and paying for these services.

1 What are the benefits of receiving care in the home?
2 What can a physician learn in a home visit that will provide better assessment information than that which is obtained during an office visit?
3 Spencer's previous medical experiences have mainly occurred in the emergency department. How could continuity of care benefit his healthcare and family?

## Additional scene

a (1:30:20–1:31:30). Carol phones home while she is away on a brief trip. She is overjoyed to hear from her mother that Spencer is out playing soccer and that he has scored a goal.

# Diabetes

◆ *Steel Magnolias* (Sally Field, Dolly Parton, Shirley MacLaine, Olympia Dukakis, Julia Roberts, Tom Skerritt). This movie takes place in the South in the 1980s. Shelby (Julia Roberts) is planning her wedding with the help of her mother, M'Lynn (Sally Field), and her father, Drum (Tom Skerritt). Shelby has diabetes. Much of the activity occurs in the beauty salon owned by a family friend, Truvy (Dolly Parton). It is in the salon that the truth is told and family secrets are revealed.

a (0:18:37–0:28:02). At the beauty salon, Shelby, her mother and their friends are getting their hair done in preparation for the wedding. Shelby states that 'I just like the idea of growing old with somebody.' She begins to show symptoms of hypoglycemia. Her mother and friends quickly come to her aid, which she resists and resents.

1 What family dynamics are revealed in this scene?
2 How would you describe the mother–daughter relationship?
3 What is the impact of diabetes throughout the family life cycle?
4 How does the age of the person affect the reaction to the illness?
5 How does diabetes affect the relationship between mother and daughter?
6 What kind of coping mechanisms do individuals with diabetes develop?
7 How does diabetes affect significant relationships outside the family unit?

b (0:52:30–0:59:00). M'Lynn and Shelby are talking in the kitchen when Shelby reveals that she is going to have a baby. M'Lynn reacts with fear, anger and disapproval.

1   What prompts M'Lynn's reaction?
2   What are the risks associated with pregnancy and diabetes?
3   How would you counsel a diabetic patient with regard to her desire to bear a child?
4   How does the mother's reaction affect Shelby?
5   What were Shelby's hopes in sharing this information with her mother?

## Progression of the disease

◆ *Steel Magnolias* (Sally Field, Dolly Parton, Shirley Maclaine, Olympia Dukakis, Julie Roberts, Tom Skerritt). See previous section on diabetes for movie description.

a (1:06:52–1:15:10). This scene takes place in the beauty salon. Shelby decides to get her nails done and Truvy (Dolly Parton) notices the severe scarring on her arms. Shelby and M'Lynn acknowledge that Shelby is on dialysis and needs a kidney transplant.

1   As a family physician, how would you counsel this patient about the physical challenges that she is facing?
2   What anticipatory guidance could you offer to both Shelby and her mother?
3   What aspects of the mother–daughter relationship are revealed in this scene? How would you interpret Shelby's desire for independence and her intense need for her mother's approval?

b (1:18:04–1:18:58). M'Lynn is donating a kidney to Shelby. It is the night before Shelby is scheduled for surgery and the family is playing cards.

1   What does this scene reveal about individual and family coping mechanisms?
2   How would you counsel a family about organ donation? How would you prepare a family to face the possibility of organ rejection?
3   What psychological reactions could you expect if the transplant does not work?
4   How would you counsel a family about feelings of failure and loss related to organ rejection?
5   What are the advantages and disadvantages of family-related organ donation?

◆ *Soul Food* (Vanessa Williams, Vivica A Fox, Nia Long, Brandon Hammond, Irma P Hall). The matriarch of the Joseph family, Big Mama, has diabetes which she has not been controlling, despite family admonitions.

a (0:21:14–0:22:10). Big Mama is not doing well. She is told that her leg may need to be amputated.

b (0:31:50–0:34:34). Big Mama is getting her leg amputated. Her family is in the waiting room. She has a stroke during surgery and then falls into a coma.

1   What are the challenges of diabetic management?

2 How would you work with a patient who has been non-adherent?

3 How important is it to screen for depression in diabetic patients?

4 How can the patient's family be involved in the treatment plan?

5 What is the role of the family in fostering or hindering compliance with medical regimens?

6 What is the role of cultural, ethnic and religious beliefs in coping with chronic illness?

### Additional scenes

a *Steel Magnolias* (1:26:50–1:33:25). This shows a series of events ranging from Shelby playing with her baby and collapsing, to the family's decision to turn off Shelby's respirator.

b *Steel Magnolias* (1:35:28–1:45:46). This scene takes place at the cemetery where Shelby has been buried. This powerful scene portrays M'Lynn's devastation and reaction to the loss of her daughter.

## Stroke

◆ *Flawless* (Robert De Niro, Philip Seymour Hoffman). Walter Koontz (Robert De Niro) was once a hero cop and is now a security guard who lives in a run-down tenement building. One night when he responds to cries for help in his apartment building, he suffers a stroke. Depressed and reluctant, he receives rehabilitation. His physical therapist recommends music and voice lessons to help his speech. Since he does not want to go out, he seeks help from a musically inclined neighbor (Philip Seymour Hoffman) who works as a female impersonator and whom he dislikes. These two people form an unlikely friendship and come to better understand each other's world.

a. (0:15:10–0:15:48). Koontz is found lying on the staircase of his apartment building. He is taken to the hospital and told by the physician that he has had a stroke and has some right-sided paralysis.

b (0:17:10–0:19:54). Koontz is discharged from the hospital and refuses an offer of a ride home. He mumbles in slurred speech that he is okay. We see him out in his neighborhood where people note his changed appearance. An old woman in his building asks why he is walking 'so funny.'

c (0:22:11–0:24:05). The physician visits Koontz at his apartment. She expresses concern that he has not come for his appointments and is housebound. She offers home physical therapy.

1 What are the risk factors for stroke?

2 What other diagnosis does this patient have and how is it impacting his rehabilitation?

3 In these scenes we see Koontz refuse contact with friends and isolate himself. What advice would you give to a family member who expressed these concerns about a relative?

4 What treatment would you recommend for Koontz?

5 What community resources are available for stroke patients and their families?

# Caregiving and caregiver burnout[1]

◆ *Marvin's Room* (Meryl Streep, Leonardo DiCaprio, Diane Keaton, Robert De Niro). Bessy (Diane Keaton) is the sole caregiver for her father, Marvin, who has been bed-bound and demented for quite a while. Things change when Bessy is diagnosed with leukemia. At this point her estranged sister, Lee, re-enters her life with her two sons.

a (0:09:56–0:13:31). Bessy's aunt is caring for Marvin while Bessy is at the doctor's office. Bessy returns to find out that her aunt did not remember to give Marvin his medication. He is demented, and Bessy takes game dice out of his mouth. We see that the aunt is afraid to be alone with Marvin. Bessy gently calms her father by using a hand mirror to create moving reflections on the wall.

1 Caregivers are hidden patients as well. How can we better attend to their needs when we see the people they care for in the office?
2 What are common signs of caregiver strain?
3 What recommendations would you give to caregivers regarding their own needs?
4 What are the available resources for caregivers?
5 Bessy is able to calm her father. What are other ways in which a caregiver learns to deal with the catastrophic reactions of dementia? How can they teach those skills to other 'substitute' caregivers?
6 What is the role of respite care? How would you encourage a caregiver to consider respite services?

# Truth-telling

◆ *Marvin's Room* (Meryl Streep, Leonardo DiCaprio, Diane Keaton, Robert De Niro). See previous section on caregiving and caregiver burnout for movie description.

a (0:25:38–0:28:06). Bessy's aunt, Ruth, visits her in the hospital during her chemotherapy. Bessy asks for her father and discovers that Ruth has not been honest with him about her absence from home. Ruth has told Marvin that Bessy is just busy in the next room. She also pretends not to notice the home health nurse who visits, saying 'I pretend that she is not real.' Bessy is upset at the prospect that her father may be further confused.

1 How would you respond to a patient like Ruth who is not truthful about the whereabouts and/or condition of another family member?
2 How would you respond to a family member who asked you not to disclose the diagnosis to the patient?
3 Bessy is still caring for others while also taking care of herself. What advice could you give an individual/family in this situation?

## Reference

1. Parks SM, Novielli KD. A practical guide to caring for caregivers. *Am Fam Physician* 2000; **62**: 2613–22.

# Chapter 8

# Geriatric medicine

*Wadie Najm and Patricia Lenahan*

As medical sciences are achieving great advances in healthcare, and people become more health conscious, life expectancy has increased dramatically. Despite these advances, a higher prevalence of cancer, chronic medical conditions (e.g. osteoarthritis, hypertension) and age-specific health concerns (e.g. medications, function, depression) continue to impact on the care of the older person. Less than 5% of the elderly reside in nursing homes. The majority of them function physically well on their own and are cared for in outpatient settings by primary care physicians. Healthcare providers must pay particular attention to elements of the social history (e.g. living arrangements, financial status, elder abuse, caregiver stress), functional ability, cognitive status (e.g. memory, depression, anxiety, substance abuse), pain assessment, medication review, nutrition, immunizations, patient values, and advanced directives for long-term and end-of-life care. The following movies provide a platform for teachers to introduce these topics and lead students and residents in discussion.

## Retirement

◆ *About Schmidt* (Jack Nicholson, Kathy Bates, Hope Davis, Dermot Mulroney). Warren Schmidt (Jack Nicholson) is an actuarial agent facing retirement, the sudden unexpected death of his wife and an estranged relationship with his daughter, who is planning her wedding. He sets out on a journey of self-discovery and is aided by his correspondence with a young boy whom he has 'adopted' through an international children's aid program.

a (0:02:10–0:06:00). Warren and his wife are seen at his retirement party. A friend who is already retired asks Warren how he feels about 'these young punks' taking over their jobs. The friend comments that what is meaningful to him is that Warren has devoted his life to a career and raising a family. He adds that if he has done his job, then he is a rich man.

1 What is the significance of work in an individual's assessment of self-worth?
2 Freud said that the two most important things in a person's life are to love and to work. If that is true, how can an individual prepare for retirement?
3 Imagine your own retirement. What factors would affect your ability to adapt to this life-stage change?

b (0:09:10–0:11:17). This scene finds Schmidt on his first day of retirement, waking up as usual and sitting in his office doing word puzzles. He hears a horn honking and goes outside. His wife has fixed breakfast in the motor caravan to see what it will be like when they travel. She toasts him and says 'Here's to a whole new chapter.'

1  What stereotypes of aging and post-retirement life does this scene portray?
2  The Schmidts appear to be a financially stable couple. What issues confront aging couples who have fewer resources?

c  (0:18:00–0:22:28). Schmidt is in his office writing a letter to his foster child. He focuses on the physical changes of aging and describes himself as a 66-year-old man with sagging skin, veins on his legs and hair in his ears, and that he can't believe it is him. He then asks who is the old woman who lives in his house. He has become more irritated with his wife since retirement, and complains about the way she sits and the way she smells.

1  What factors influence successful adaptation to retirement?
2  What is the effect of retirement on marital relationships?

# Loss of spouse

◆ *About Schmidt* (Jack Nicholson, Kathy Bates, Hope Davis, Dermot Mulroney). See previous section on retirement for movie description.

a  (0:25:25–0:29:45). Schmidt comes into the house and finds his wife sprawled on the kitchen floor. He tries to revive her, without success. The scene shifts to the coroner removing Helen's body from the house and to the funeral director, who discusses burial costs. At the cemetery, the minister tells Warren that anger is okay and God can handle anger.

1  What are the risk factors associated with the loss of a spouse in aging couples?

b  (0:42:12–0:45:45). Warren talks about being alone in this big house. He is in his pajamas eating in front of the television. He comments that the actuarial tables' statistics predict he has a 73% chance of dying in nine years now that his wife has died. He decides that he should make the best of the time he has left and then falls asleep in front of the television. The scene shifts to two weeks later. He is still in his pajamas, the house is a mess and he acknowledges that he misses some meals. He puts on his wife's cold cream, smells her perfume and stares at her clothing.

1  Discuss bereavement. What are the typical stages that a bereaved person experiences?
2  What is the role of the physician in caring for a bereaved older adult?
3  What risk factors must you consider?
4  What anticipatory guidance can a physician offer a bereaved patient?

c  (1:54:55–1:55:58). Warren enters the house and says that he is weak and a failure. He wonders what difference his life has made to anyone, and that once everyone who knows him has died, it will be as if he never existed.

1  What factors contribute to successful aging?
2  What is the significance of *life review therapy* in the lives of older adults? How can it be used to promote adaptation to life changes?

3  According to Erikson, what life stage is Warren experiencing? What are the developmental tasks of this stage?

## Functional assessment

◆ *Dad* (Jack Lemmon, Ted Danson, Olympia Dukakis). This movie addresses the dynamics of family life, marriage and the challenges of old age.

a  (0:09:32–0:14:47). In this clip, John Tremont (Ted Danson) is an investment banker who is called to Los Angeles when his mother, Bette (Olympia Dukakis), suffers a heart attack. While she is in hospital, John stays with his father, Jake (Jack Lemmon), whom he has not seen for two years. After growing completely dependent on his wife for years, Jake seems helpless and unable to care for himself.

1  Who are the caregivers of the elderly? Discuss the impact of role reversal (i.e. adult children having to 'parent' their elderly parents) on family life.
2  What are the basic functions needed for an elderly person to live independently in the home or in the community?
3  How do you screen or evaluate the activities of daily living (ADL) and the instrumental activities of daily living (IADL)?
4  What can be done to allow the elderly with limited ADL to remain at home?

## Mental status testing and medical interventions

◆ *Iris* (Judi Dench, Jim Broadbent, Kate Winslet, Hugh Bonneville). Based on John Bagley's book, *Elegy for Iris,* this film recounts the life of Iris Murdoch (a British author and philosopher) and her husband (also an author) as they cope with the onset and progression of Iris's Alzheimer's disease.

a  (0:25:57–0:31:10). When Iris is unable to answer the physician's question 'Who is the Prime Minister?', he turns to John and asks him if this happens often. The doctor discusses specialists, magnetic resonance imaging (MRI) and other medical interventions with John. Iris overhears their conversation and is frightened. She says that she feels as if she is going into the darkness, and John emphasizes that she must keep talking and working. Iris confuses 'God' and 'dog' on a test, and John, who is in denial, tells the doctor that she is just tired.

1  Do anxiety and fatigue affect the outcome of mental status testing?
2  What do you think of John's advice to Iris to keep on talking and working?
3  How does denial impact on the identification and treatment of dementia?

## Medications and cognition

◆ *Dad* (Jack Lemmon, Ted Danson, Olympia Dukakis). See previous section on functional assessment for movie description.

a  (0:47:00–0:56:38). In this clip, Jake is diagnosed with cancer. His son John asks the doctor not to divulge the diagnosis of cancer to him. Jake undergoes surgery and is experiencing delirium (*see* Chapter 7 for another clip which addresses truth telling).

1  To maintain one's ethical responsibilities, what steps should be taken when the family does not want the physician to divulge the diagnosis to the patient?
2  What are the specific challenges encountered by the elderly when undergoing surgery?
3  What strategies can physicians use to communicate the diagnosis of delirium? How can physicians best manage delirium? How does one differentiate delirium from dementia?
4  How does one ensure that the medical community will comply with a patient's wishes for care (discuss appropriate timing for completing advance directives)?

## Hospital discharge and planning

◆ *Dad* (Jack Lemmon, Ted Danson, Olympia Dukakis). See earlier section on functional assessment for movie description.

a  (0:56:38–0:59:52). In this scene, Jake's doctor discharges him home while he is still in a delirious state.

1  What steps should be taken to ensure the safe and appropriate discharge of an elderly patient?
2  What support services are available to elderly patients and their family members in your community?

b  (0:25:06–0:26:40). In this clip, John develops a plan which allows his father to participate in the housework.

1  Discuss what can be done to allow elderly people to stay at home despite their physical or mental limitations.

## Home safety and future planning

◆ *Folks* (Tom Selleck, Don Ameche). John Aldrich (Tom Selleck), preoccupied with his busy life, has not seen his parents for several years. He travels to Miami following his mother's hospitalization to find that his father, Harry Aldrich (Don Ameche), is having memory problems.

a  (0:41:30–0:45:00). In this scene, John's parents come to live with him and his family. His father, Harry, has to deal with his new surroundings.

1  Discuss some of the changes that can be made to prevent injury at home.
2  What topics should be discussed with the family members and/or the caregiver of the patient when dementia is diagnosed (e.g. Durable Power of Attorney Health Care (DPAHC), Medi-Alert bracelet, medications, driving, caregiver stress, support group).

## Falls

◆ *In the Bedroom* (Sissy Spacek, Tom Wilkinson, Marisa Tomei). Although this is mainly a film that addresses family violence, family relationships and coping with loss, it provides a brief yet excellent aging-related clip.

a (0:13:04–0:13:56). Mr Adamson is reading a children's magazine while he and his wife are waiting to see Dr Fowler (Tom Wilkinson). In the examination room, Mrs Adamson helps her husband to put his shirt on. She tells Dr Fowler that he was okay the day before, but he fell today. She also says that her husband has fallen twice and is getting weaker. She continues, 'My husband said that he didn't want to live if he couldn't work.' At the end of their visit, Mr Adamson asks about the health of Dr Fowler's father, who has been dead for several years. His wife is very apologetic.

1   What factors contribute to falls in the elderly?
2   What outcomes are linked to falls?
3   What aspects of a physical exam should the doctor focus on to address balance and home safety issues?
4   How can the elderly seniors reduce their risk of falling? What can they do if they do fall?
5   What constitutes 'fear of falling phobia'?

## Nursing home placement

◆ *Marvin's Room* (Meryl Streep, Leonardo DiCaprio, Diane Keaton, Robert De Niro). Bessy (Diane Keaton) is the sole caregiver for her father, Marvin, who has been bed-bound and demented for quite a while. Things change when Bessy is diagnosed with leukemia. Her estranged sister, Lee, then re-enters her life with her two sons.

a (0:55:04–0:58:35). Lee and Bessy tour a nursing home for their father. Bessy reflects that 'Dad would never have put Mom in a place like this.' The sisters argue about why Lee can't take their father and Aunt Ruth to live with her.

1   What are some of the financial, emotional, geographic and family issues associated with nursing home placement?
2   What advice would you give a family member regarding this decision? What if a family member asked you what you would do if the patient were your own parent?
3   Have any of you been personally involved in such a decision?

## Dementia

### Diagnosing dementia

◆ *Folks* (Tom Selleck, Don Ameche). See earlier section on home safety and future planning for movie description.

a (0:30:39–0:33:30). In this scene, John takes his mother home from the hospital, where they find that her house has burned down because John left his father home alone.

1   Discuss the most common forms of dementia.
2   Discuss the early signs and symptoms of dementia and Alzheimer's disease.
3   Discuss the different office tests that can be used to screen for and/or diagnose dementia.

## Early onset of dementia

◆ *Iris* (Judi Dench, Jim Broadbent, Kate Winslet, Hugh Bonneville). See earlier
section on mental status testing and medical interventions for movie description.

a (0:17:04–0:17:51). Here we see that writing is becoming harder for Iris, and she
has difficulty spelling.

b (0:24:00–25:50). Iris is giving a televised interview and loses her train of
thought. She returns home from the studio not knowing why she was there,
and then asks her husband about a person who has been dead for some time.

1  What factors may have contributed to Iris's reactions at the television studio?
2  What is the importance of maintaining a routine and schedule for a patient
   with Alzheimer's disease?
3  What is the significance for Iris, as an author, of having difficulty in spelling
   words?

## Middle stages of Alzheimer's disease

◆ *Iris* (Judi Dench, Jim Broadbent, Kate Winslet, Hugh Bonneville). See earlier
section on mental status testing and medical interventions for movie description.

a (0:32:50–0:34:50). Iris answers the door and is frightened because she could
not identify the postman. She follows John around the house, repeating 'It's only
the postman.' He becomes irritated with her repetition.

1  What is the cause of the patient's fear?
2  How does her repetition of words and phrases help to alleviate this fear?
3  What is the impact on the caregiver?

# Caregiver strain

◆ *Iris* (Judi Dench, Jim Broadbent, Kate Winslet, Hugh Bonneville). See earlier
section on mental status testing and medical interventions for movie description.

a (0:44:45–0:45:10). Iris is yelling for help and John is trying to help her.

b (0:59:58–1:02:20). Iris is singing and wandering around the house during the
night. John gets up to help her to get back into bed.

1  What is the impact of caregiver strain for both the patient and the caregiver?
2  What advice would you offer patients and caregivers to help to ease the
   caregiver burden?
3  What is the role of caregiver support groups?

# Late stages and death

◆ *Iris* (Judi Dench, Jim Broadbent, Kate Winslet, Hugh Bonneville). See earlier
section on mental status testing and medical interventions for movie description.

a (1:20:05–1:21:50). Iris becomes hysterical after a friend's funeral. She jumps out of the car and John chases after her. Iris, struggling for words, tells John that she loves him. Later, their physician makes a home visit and tells John that it is time to place Iris in an extended care facility (ECF). While the doctor is there, he also checks on John's health.

b (1:21:50–1:24:55). The driver comes to collect Iris, but John cannot get her off the stairs. John holds Iris's hand on the way to the ECF. We see the facility as John sees it and observe Iris dancing in the hall. Later, John is with Iris as she dies.

1 How does caregiving affect health?
2 What factors contribute to a spouse's/family's decision to place their loved one in a nursing home?
3 What supports can be offered to the caregiver after the death of a loved one?
4 How can physicians assist caregivers in resuming their lives after their caregiving roles have ended?

# Chapter 9

# Life threatening illness/end of life

*Joseph Kertesz and Anna Pavlov*

Addressing the emotional needs of the individual at the end of life is one of the most challenging tasks faced by any physician. In such situations, physicians can no longer rely primarily on their medical knowledge, which is geared towards diagnosis and treatment. Instead, they have to depend on their *interpersonal skills and sensitivity* in order to empathize with and provide comfort for those who are dying as well as their families. Cinemeducation is a wonderful way to educate physicians about the magnitude of emotions that arise during these most difficult of circumstances. It can also help to highlight the practical issues that face a patient and their family at the end of life, and how physicians can best manage these issues.

## Giving bad news

◆ *Terms of Endearment* (Shirley MacLaine, Debra Winger, Jack Nicholson, Jeff Daniels). This movie skillfully examines the enmeshment between Aurora (Shirley MacLaine) and her daughter Emma (Debra Winger). Emma's father died while she was young and she has no siblings. As the film progresses, the viewer experiences the strength of this mother–daughter bond. The movie culminates with Emma's battle with a terminal illness.

a (1:33:40–1:34:42). Emma and her daughter are at the doctor's office getting flu shots. The physician discovers lumps in Emma's armpit.

b (1:35:52–1:36:20). The physician delivers the news that Emma has a malignancy.

c (1:44:05–1:45:12). The oncologist tells Emma that her cancer is non-responsive to treatment. She begins to realize the gravity of her circumstances and wonders what will happen to her children. The physician's discomfort in this situation is obvious.

1  What stages of grief did you observe in Emma throughout these clips?
2  What physician behaviors did you observe?
3  Were there any skills that you would utilize as a physician that you did not observe in these scenes? What would you have done differently?
4  What special needs do children have when a parent is dying?
5  What role do you think spirituality plays in dealing with end-of-life issues?

◆ *Wit* (Emma Thompson, Christopher Lloyd). Vivian Bearing PhD (Emma Thompson) is an 'uncompromising' English professor diagnosed with stage 4 ovarian cancer. Throughout the film she chronicles and provides commentary on her devastating illness and experimental treatment, her reaction to health-care providers and the demoralizing aspects of medical care.

a (0:00:33–0:04:11). In this scene, Dr Bearing is given her cancer diagnosis and presented with treatment options. She is told by the oncologist, 'You must be very tough. Do you think you can be very tough?'.

1 How does this physician go about giving bad news? Is this portrayal an exaggeration?
2 How does this scene illustrate the importance of taking into account patients' level of education when giving medical information? How would you have phrased things differently?
3 What feedback would you give the oncologist about this encounter? *Suggestion:* role play an alternative approach.
4 What are some key elements of giving bad news?
5 What message about emotions and coping with cancer would *you* want to give the patient? What information would *you* provide up front?

## Healthcare provider reactions to end-of-life issues

◆ *Life as a House* (Kevin Kline, Kristin Scott Thomas, Hayden Christensen, Mary Steenburgen). This is the story of an architect, George (Kevin Kline), who learns that he has four months to live. Up until this time he has lived a solitary existence and alienated most of the people in his life. When he learns that he is terminally ill, he decides to reconnect with his estranged son Sam (Hayden Christensen). He tells Sam, who is in the throes of being a rebellious teenager, that he wants his assistance in building a house. George does not reveal his underlying motivation for this house-building project. The film includes many interesting depictions of family dynamics as George pursues his house-building dream with Sam and his ex-wife Robin (Kristin Scott Thomas). The impact of George's disease on all involved becomes obvious later in the movie after George reveals that he is dying.

a (0:10:00–0:22:42). In these clips George is first seen coming out of his office building having just been fired. He passes out, is taken to the hospital and is told that he has a terminal illness with a life expectancy of four months. The next scene shows him talking with the nurse about his feelings. The nurse demonstrates great sensitivity and compassion. The last scene closes with George revealing that he is scared.

1 What emotions, other than fear, do you think that George is experiencing?
2 What skills do you observe in the nurse?
3 Have you been in a similar situation with a terminally ill patient? How did you handle it? What impact did it have on you?

◆ *Wit* (Emma Thompson, Christopher Lloyd). See previous section on giving bad news for movie description.

a (0:31:10–0:35:00). Teaching rounds at the bedside.

1 What aspects of the case presentation are valued in medical education? Do they necessarily impress the patient?

2   What are some ways for bedside rounds to be both a good teaching experience *and* a good experience for the patient?
3   Is empathy demonstrated in the encounter?
4   What can you do when you have 'compassion fatigue'?
5   How common are depression and anxiety in cancer patients?

## Family reactions to end of life

◆   *Life as a House* (Kevin Kline, Kristin Scott Thomas, Hayden Christensen, Mary Steenburgen). See previous section on healthcare provider reactions for movie description.

a   (1:36:40–1:42:35). In this clip we see George informing Sam that he has a terminal illness. George has already accepted his fate. The power in this scene lies in Sam's reaction, which reveals a full range of emotions that are entirely understandable.

1   Describe the emotions that you witness in Sam.
2   What other emotions have you seen family members experience after they have been given this kind of tragic information? Are there cultural differences in family reactions to the end of life?
3   What skills does a physician need in order to help patients and their families in these circumstances?
4   What is the role of support systems in helping individuals and their families to deal with end-of-life issues?

◆   *Behind the Red Door* (Kiefer Sutherland, Kyra Sedgwick, Stockard Channing). This movie is about a family that has been split apart by a physically abusive father. We pick up the story when the children are adults. They are trying to move on with their lives, but continue to be hampered by past demons. The daughter, Natalie (Kyra Sedgwick), is a photographer in New York who has not seen her brother, Roy (Kiefer Sutherland), for ten years. Their last meeting was when their mother was murdered. Although many suspect that it was their father who killed her, this was never proved. Roy, who still lives in Boston, is very successful, gay and, unbeknownst to Natalie, has AIDS. They are brought together when Natalie is contracted to shoot Roy's latest advertising campaign.

a   (0:18:00–0:24:00). In this scene Natalie is trying to leave her brother's home. Her work has been completed and she no longer wants to spend time with him. He persuades her to stay for breakfast, and then tells her that he is sick and wants her help.

b   (0:26:40–0:30:15). Roy is now in the hospital, spiking a fever. This is Natalie's first experience of trying to give him assistance while he is ill. The nurse is there briefly but then leaves. Natalie and Roy begin to talk about death as punishment and how they would like to know about their own death.

1   Describe Natalie's reaction to the news that her brother is seriously ill.
2   How do you explain Natalie's fixation with Roy's stopping smoking?

3 How might the reaction of an adult sibling to another adult sibling's terminal illness be different from that of other family members?
4 What was your reaction to Roy's perception that death might be his punishment? How common is this perception in AIDS patients? How would you 'disabuse' a patient of this notion?
5 If you could, would you want to know how and when you were going to die? Why or why not?

## Pediatric illness

◆ *Lorenzo's Oil* (Susan Sarandon, Nick Nolte, Zack O'Malley Greenberg). This is the cinematic adaptation of a true story about Lorenzo (Zack O'Malley Greenberg), a boy with adrenoleukodystrophy, a rare, terminal and untreatable illness at the time, and his parents' (Nick Nolte, Susan Sarandon) fight to prolong their child's life against all odds.

a (0:08:05–0:19:08). These scenes portray the progression of events from Lorenzo's early symptoms to his parents being told of his diagnosis and prognosis. He initially shows signs of aggression, poor balance and hearing loss. The scene in which his parents receive the news of their son's condition is a powerful depiction of a mother and father's worst nightmare.

1 What would it be like to hear that your child is dying?
2 What stages of grief did you view the parents going through?
3 What was your reaction to Dr Junalung's style? What did he do well? What could he have done differently? *Suggestion:* role play an alternative approach.

◆ *Terms of Endearment* (Shirley MacLaine, Debra Winger, Jack Nicholson, Jeff Daniels). See earlier section on giving bad news for movie description.

a (1:57:05–2:02:18). In this scene Emma says goodbye to the boys and explains what they should expect for the future.

1 When and how would you suggest that terminally ill patients inform their children about their prognosis?
2 How do you cope with your emotional reactions to sad outcomes in medicine?

## Patient's perspective of end of life

◆ *Wit* (Emma Thompson, Christopher Lloyd). See earlier section on giving bad news' for movie description.

a (0:04:20–0:06:20). This scene contains a soliloquy describing the patient's reaction to the diagnosis of cancer and her experience of doctor–patient interactions.

1 Did you learn anything from this scene that you had not previously considered about the experience of cancer patients?
2 What can be done to minimize some of the issues so vividly captured by Dr Bearing (e.g. other ways to ask 'How are you feeling?')?

# Code status

◆ *Wit* (Emma Thompson, Christopher Lloyd). See earlier section on giving bad news for movie description.

a (1:00:16–1:10:50). The nurse is at the patient's bedside in the middle of the night. She provides the patient with emotional support in coping with her uncertainties and talks with her about code status and DNR (do not resuscitate) orders.

1   While a nurse would not typically initiate a discussion about code status, highlight the strengths of the way in which this healthcare professional discusses a difficult topic.
2   Does this scene give you any new ideas of ways to discuss the topic?
3   How might the patient's experience have differed if she had had a family physician?
4   What are the challenges of discussing code status with patients and with families? What obstacles/challenges have you experienced?
5   What are common patient and family concerns in designating DNR and in agreeing to hospice care?

# Finding a bone-marrow donor

◆ *Marvin's Room* (Meryl Streep, Leonardo DiCaprio, Diane Keaton, Robert De Niro, Hume Cronyn). Bessy (Diane Keaton) is the sole caregiver for her father, Marvin (Hume Cronyn), who has been bed-bound and demented for quite a while. Things change when Bessy is diagnosed with leukemia. Her estranged sister, Lee (Meryl Streep), then re-enters her life with her two sons.

a (0:52:47–054:20). Lee asks Bessy about her prognosis on the 'off chance that you can't find a donor.' The physician explains the possible outcomes and says, 'eventually you'll have to find a full-time nurse to help you.' Lee does not seem to hear this, and replies 'She's going to be fine.'

1   What are some of the emotional issues that come into play when seeking family members who could be potential bone-marrow donors?

# Part III

Adult diagnostic categories

Chapter 10

# Post-traumatic stress disorder

*Joseph Kertesz, Patricia Lenahan and Robert Tran*

Post-traumatic stress disorder (PTSD) is rarely easy to identify in primary care settings, and often goes undiagnosed. It is common for individuals with PTSD to have multiple and frequent medical complaints. This leads the primary care clinician to pursue medical work-ups when, in fact, the physical distress is psychological in origin.

One of the main barriers to the identification of PTSD by physicians is their lack of a point of reference with regard to this disorder. Unless they have personally experienced trauma, they are often unable to fully appreciate the psychological impact of this disorder. A case in point is the fact that many of the more than 20 million people who emigrate to the USA each year come from war-torn nations where they may have experienced violence in their home and community. A substantial percentage of these refugees have experienced or witnessed numerous catastrophes and atrocities, such as famine, war, rape and repression, over an extended period of time. PTSD also frequently occurs as a result of more commonplace events that are outside the experience of many healthcare professionals, such as robberies and motor-vehicle accidents.

Film clips can provide a means for physicians to begin to realize and visualize the magnitude of the emotional trauma for the individual, and may ultimately assist in facilitating better diagnosis and treatment of this disorder.

## PTSD secondary to rape

◆ *Things Behind the Sun* (Kim Dickens, Gabriel Mann, Don Cheadle, Eric Stoltz). This ShowTime original movie addresses the long-term impact of a gang rape on both the victim, Sherry (Kim Dickens), and one of the perpetrators of the rape, Owen (Gabriel Mann). Sherry was in her early teens when the rape occurred, as was Owen, who was forced by his brother to participate in the rape. When Owen and Sherry are adults they re-establish a relationship through a series of events. The actual events of the rape unfold through a series of flashbacks in the minds of both Owen and Sherry.

a (1:08:10–1:10:18). In this clip, Owen and Sherry are talking in Owen's hotel room. Sherry decides to take a shower, and seeing the soap in the soap holder causes her to have a flashback. The soap is similar to the one that was located in the room where she was raped, and it brings back traumatic memories of that event. The flashback paralyzes her and then terrorizes her until she finally collapses.

b (1:42:10–1:47:05). Trying to confront her demons, Sherry goes back to the house where she was raped. The owner of the house realizes the power that the house has over her and, fortunately for her, welcomes her in. The scene portrays great intensity and the beginning of Sherry's healing process as she recalls the memories of being attacked there. This scene is also a wonderful example of the startle response that is often seen in PTSD.

c (1:12:55–1:14:20). Owen is in his car and has a flashback of the rape. Note that Owen's trauma trigger is the ceiling fan.

1 What would it be like to have an object, benign to the rest of the world, trigger such intense terror and memories that it causes a person to be unable to function?
2 What do you think is the long-term impact of experiencing trauma such as rape?
3 What are the skills needed by a physician in order to encourage a person to reveal these personal nightmares?
4 How might a patient exhibit signs of PTSD in the office (e.g. jumpiness, sudden and unexplained change in affect, dissociation)? What patient behaviors and mannerisms might suggest to you the possibility of PTSD (e.g. refusal to have a Pap smear)?

## PTSD secondary to a motor-vehicle accident

◆ *The Waterdance* (Eric Stoltz, William Forsythe, Wesley Snipes, Helen Hunt). This film follows the lives of several men at a rehabilitation facility who have spinal cord injuries. *The Waterdance* focuses on the patients and their families as they try to adapt to all of the life changes that occur as a consequence of their injuries.

a (0:33:48–0:34:00). At the rehabilitation center, Bloss (William Forsythe), an argumentative man who was hit by a car, is drinking with visitors who spur him on to telephone the man who caused the accident that has left him paralyzed. Bloss then asks the man how he feels about running over an innocent person, and mentions that a hefty lawsuit is in the making.

b (0:50:20–0:51:02). Bloss, his lawyer and his mother are on the street corner where the accident occurred. The lawyer asks Bloss to recount the details of the accident. His mother asks Bloss if he is okay, because he begins to look more and more distressed. He asks if they can talk about this in a restaurant. Finally, when he says he has to find a bathroom, they leave the scene.

1 What symptoms might Bloss be experiencing?
2 What differentiates PTSD from acute stress disorder?
3 After seeing Bloss's symptoms, would it be possible to make a diagnosis of adjustment disorder?
4 How might the matter of litigation affect the way in which you assessed or managed Bloss's care?
5 Do the patient's lifestyle and prior behavior affect the way in which you regard him and/or handle his situation?

# PTSD secondary to political torture

◆ *Down Came a Blackbird* (Laura Dern, Vanessa Redgrave, Raul Julia). Journalist Helen McNulty (Laura Dern) is traveling in an unidentified Central American country with her photographer boyfriend (Jay Saunders) when they observe, and photograph, a political rally that turns deadly. They are subsequently kidnapped, tortured, and Helen's boyfriend is murdered. A year later, Helen is back in the USA pitching a story to her editor. She wants to interview a psychiatrist who runs a clinic for survivors of torture. Helen goes to the clinic as a writer, unwilling to admit that she, too, is a survivor of torture.

a (0:06:00–0:06:53, 0:12:40–0:15:36). Helen is in Portland one year after the incident. The scene focuses on the disarray of her apartment. Helen is having a flashback of making love with her boyfriend while drinking, popping pills, looking at her journal and hugging a photograph of him.

1 What is the impact of untreated PTSD?
2 With what kinds of symptoms do you suppose Helen presented to her physician in order to obtain the medications that she is taking?

b (0:19:25–0:22:28). Dr Lenke (Vanessa Redgrave) examines Helen and asks her if she has any physical complaints or injuries. She also asks Helen what medication she is taking that is causing her pulse rate to be so high. She gently probes Helen for answers and continues to ask for all the medications until Helen admits to using sleeping pills.

1 How does 'self-medication' affect the overall treatment process?
2 If medications are misused in order to numb feelings and repress memories, what effect will their removal have on the therapeutic process?

c (0:29:07–0:32:04). Helen is having a nightmare and awakens out of breath. She goes out to the patio to have a cigarette, and meets Thomas, a new patient. He does not sleep well either, saying that he reads until dawn and then falls asleep for just an hour or two. Helen tells him that she prefers 'chemicals.'

1 How do sleep disturbance and insomnia further complicate the patient's functioning?
2 How would you manage insomnia in a patient with PTSD?

d (0:32:53–0:38:04). Dr Lenke begins a therapy session by asking everyone to introduce themselves and indicate that they are survivors of torture. The group members are from a variety of cultures and include a Greek, an African and an Eastern European. Dr Lenke discusses the similarities of all torture survivor stories, and gently encourages Helen to acknowledge that she is a survivor of torture and to share her story.

1 What are the universal aspects of torture and survival?
2 What common themes could be seen among this disparate group of people?

e (0:55:00–0:56:40). Dr Lenke meets with Myrna (Sarita Choundhury) and tries to engage her in conversation. She acknowledges that she had really upset Myrna the day before, but Myrna angrily responds that she cannot possibly know how she feels. Dr Lenke tells Myrna that she *can* understand. Realizing that Dr Lenke has also been victimized by torture, Myrna asks Dr Lenke to tell her about her experiences.

1 How would you interpret Dr Lenke's personal disclosure?
2 Would you consider this self-disclosure appropriate since it enhanced the therapeutic process?
3 What guidelines would you set to best maintain professional boundaries with clients?
4 How can the power of shared experience be appropriately used in therapy?

f (0:56:42–0:59:50). Dr Lenke begins a group therapy session by saying that it is normal to remember the pain and the situation that caused the pain. She discusses the olfactory element of torture and how violence can disconnect and distort any relationship. As an example, she points out that, as a result of her torture, Helen is terrified of swimming pools. Another patient grows anxious, fearing that the Greek Generals are still searching for him.

1 How can stress trigger a flashback?
2 What does a survivor of torture think and feel when a sight or smell triggers a flashback?

g (1:16:48–1:30:15). Helen is encouraged to share her experiences in this session and she reluctantly complies. Accompanied by a series of graphic flashbacks, Helen describes being gang raped and how she momentarily felt safer when a man entered the room. She describes how her captors treated her and how she had to fight for her life. Bound and gagged, she was thrown into a swimming pool, where she discovered the body of her boyfriend lying on the bottom. Helen tells the group that she felt her boyfriend was more important than she was because they killed him and not her. She was surprised that her captors released her, and she could not fathom how normal life was once she was free – no one even knew what had happened to her. Helen expresses guilt about not trying harder to find her boyfriend after she escaped.

1 Discuss the Stockholm syndrome. Does it apply in Helen's situation?
2 What is the impact of survivor guilt?
3 What treatment strategies would you employ when addressing symptoms of chronic PTSD?
4 How might Helen's prognosis and therapy have differed if she had sought treatment immediately after the trauma occurred?

## PTSD and war/forced emigration

◆ *Green Dragon* (Patrick Swayze, Forrest Whittaker, Don Duong). This is a film about the first wave of Vietnamese refugees and their initial experiences after being displaced from their country following the end of the Vietnam War. It tells the story of the relationship formed between a Vietnamese immigrant, Minh (Don Duong), and a US Marine, Sergeant Jim Lance (Patrick Swayze), in charge of the refugee camp.

a (0:01:57–0:03:31). Sounds of guns and bombs are heard. A child wakes up panting and hears sounds of helicopters as the viewer sees the reflection of a ceiling fan rotating like helicopter blades. The child walks outside and looks up at the sky.

1  What factors contribute to flashbacks?
2  How would you counsel an immigrant family about symptoms of post-traumatic stress disorder in children?

b  (0:04:00–0:08:50). In this scene, waves of refugees are walking with their suitcases and personal belongings, having just arrived at Camp Pendleton. The refugees are relocated to Quonset huts, and search for pictures of loved ones on the bulletin boards in the camp while two children search for their mother. Some individuals are in group showers, bathing with their clothes on. Others are seen exchanging rings and jewelery for American dollars.

1  In what ways does the relocation process affect physical and psychological health?
2  What do you notice about the plight of the refugees in this scene?
3  How would you intervene with refugees such as these to prevent further emotional distress?
4  What are the different ways that people migrate to the USA? What does it mean to be a refugee? How does it differ for one to emigrate as a refugee compared with other means of emigration?
5  What are some of the unique issues that physicians may encounter when caring for refugees? What issues may complicate the care of refugee populations?

# Chapter 11

# Anxiety, depression and somatoform disorders

*Matthew Alexander, Dael Waxman and Joan Simpson*

Depression is the second most common chronic diagnosis seen in primary care.[1] Anxiety disorders are also common in primary care practice. For example, individuals with panic disorder have been found to visit healthcare providers at three times the rate of other patients.[1] In fact, it is estimated that family doctors see more patients with anxiety disorder than patients with diabetes. Similarly, patients with somatization disorder, both clinical and sub-syndromal, are common. To complicate matters further, there are high rates of overlap between depression, anxiety and somatization disorder.

There is considerable evidence that up to 50% of patients with psychiatric disorders are *primarily* seen and treated by primary care physicians.[2] Such patients demonstrate greater functional impairment and higher rates of inappropriate utilization of medical resources than their non-psychiatric counterparts.[3] New pharmacologic and non-pharmacologic treatments for psychiatric disorders in primary care increase positive outcomes but make proper diagnosis of these conditions essential. However, for a variety of reasons, psychiatric disorders such as depression and anxiety tend to be under-diagnosed in primary care.[4] All of these factors taken together emphasize the importance of effective education of primary care professionals in identifying and treating depression, anxiety and somatization disorders. We have found that cinemeducation is a very useful adjunct to traditional methods of teaching learners about these important psychiatric conditions.

## Depression

### Adjustment disorder with depressed mood

◆ *An Unmarried Woman* (Jill Clayburgh, Alan Bates). This movie tells the story of Erica (Jill Clayburgh), who is forced to cope with an unexpected divorce.

a (0:34:20–0:36:18). In this scene, Erica visits her primary care physician, who makes an inappropriate 'pass' at her.

1  What aspects of adjustment disorder does this scene illustrate?
2  What other symptoms of adjustment disorder are *not* revealed in this clip?
3  What other circumstances, besides divorce, can lead patients to develop adjustment disorders?
4  What positive counseling is offered by the physician in this scene?

5 What are the current ethical guidelines on 'dating' a patient?

## Dysthymia

◆ *What's Eating Gilbert Grape?* (Johnny Depp, Leonardo DiCaprio, Darlene Cates). This movie tells the story of the Grape family, which includes Gilbert (Johnny Depp), who is 'parentified,' Arnie (Leonardo DiCaprio), who is mentally ill, and Momma (Darlene Cates), who is morbidly obese.

a (0:00:00–0:06:13). In this opening clip, Gilbert introduces us to the Grape family.

1 What are the verbal and non-verbal cues which suggest that Gilbert has dysthymia?
2 How is dysthymia different from adjustment disorder and major depression?
3 How might a dysthymic patient appear to a family doctor?
4 What are the most effective pharmacologic and non-pharmacologic treatments for dysthymia?

## Major depression

◆ *Ordinary People* (Donald Sutherland, Mary Tyler Moore). This extraordinary, award-winning movie tells the story of a family coping with the tragic death of their eldest son after a boating accident. The exact time line of the accident is unclear.

a (0:05:05–0:09:29). A succession of scenes show Conrad (Timothy Hutton), the surviving son, interacting with his family and attempting to hide his mental anguish.

1 What symptoms of major depression does Conrad demonstrate? Identify these symptoms according to their somatic, cognitive and affective aspects.
2 How does major depression differ from adjustment disorder and dysthymia?
3 Does Conrad also show symptoms of anxiety disorder? What is the comorbidity of mood disorders and anxiety disorders? Is it practical to attempt to separate these two classifications of disorder in actual practice?
4 What impact does a depressed family member have on the rest of the family?

## Mood disorder associated with a general medical condition

◆ *Safe* (Julianne Moore). This is a perplexing film about Carol White (Julianne Moore), a woman with unexplained physical symptoms who increasingly believes that she is being harmed by chemicals in the environment.

a (0:45:15–0:48:10). In this scene, Carol is writing a letter about herself to a support organization for sufferers of environmental allergies, when she is interrupted by her husband.

1 What insight did you gain from listening to White's narrative?

2 Give some examples of medical conditions that lead to secondary mood disorders.

3 How do you explain the concurrence of medical conditions with mood disorders?

4 As a healthcare professional, how can you assist individuals with this diagnosis? How do healthcare professionals sometimes inadvertently exacerbate the mood disorder of patients with general medical conditions?

5 What impact do depressed patients and those with multiple unexplained symptoms have on family members and healthcare professionals?

6 What is the role of support groups in helping individuals with mood disorders?

b (0:23:07–0:24:21). In this clip, Carol consults her primary care physician about her vague symptoms.

c (0:32:48–0:34:08). In this scene, Carol and her husband are given a referral to a psychiatrist after being pronounced physically healthy.

1 As a clinician, what does it feel like to work with people who have unexplained symptoms?

2 What are some other ways in which Carol White could have been managed?

3 What are some other medical conditions also associated with mood disorders?

# Anxiety

## Adjustment disorder with anxious mood

◆ *An Unmarried Woman* (Jill Clayburgh). See earlier section on adjustment disorder with depressed mood for movie description.

a (0:48:54–0:52:45). In this scene Erica has her first session with a therapist.

1 What are the most effective psychotherapeutic techniques for treating adjustment disorder?

2 What are the most successful ways of referring medical patients for counseling?

3 What does this therapist do that seems helpful to Erica?

4 How useful is the distinction between adjustment disorder with anxious mood and adjustment disorder with depressed mood, since anxiety and depression often coexist? Might adjustment disorder with mixed emotional features be a preferable diagnostic code?

## Panic disorder

◆ *Analyze This* (Robert De Niro, Billy Crystal). This is a hilarious movie about Paul Vitti (Robert De Niro), a powerful crime racketeer with panic disorder, and his reluctant therapist, Ben Sobel (Billy Crystal).

a (0:12:31–0:14:07). In this scene, Vitti, after nearly being killed, experiences extreme symptoms of anxiety in the presence of his mob associates.

1 What are the symptoms of panic disorder as revealed in this scene?

2  In general, how successfully do individuals hide the symptoms of a panic attack?

b  (0:14:08–0:16:27). In this scene, Vitti goes to the emergency room.

1  How do patients with panic attacks commonly 'present' to medical providers, both during and after a panic attack?
2  Why are individuals commonly ashamed of being diagnosed with mental disorders?
3  Given the stigma associated with mental illness, what is the best way to convey the diagnosis of panic disorder?
4  Distinguish between panic attacks and panic disorder.

c  (0:16:28–0:22:55). In this scene, Vitti 'arrives' for his first session with Sobel.

1  What symptoms of panic disorder are revealed in this scene?
2  What are successful pharmacologic and non-pharmacologic approaches to the treatment of panic disorder?
3  Which medical conditions mimic panic disorder? How do you distinguish these conditions from true panic disorder?

## Simple phobia

◆ *What About Bob?* (Bill Murray, Richard Dreyfuss). This dark but funny movie tells the story of Bob Wiley (Bill Murray), a highly anxious individual who invades the family life of his therapist, Dr Leo Marvin (Richard Dreyfuss).

a  (0:00:00–0:03:14). In this opening clip we see Bob attempting to make his way from his apartment to his first appointment with Dr Marvin.

1  What simple phobias are revealed in this clip?
2  What are the most common phobias seen by primary care providers?
3  What are effective treatment options for phobias?

## Generalized anxiety disorder

◆ *Hannah and Her Sisters* (Woody Allen, Mia Farrow). This is a wonderful movie about three sisters, their relationship with each other, and the men in their lives.

a  (0:14:02–0:18:19). In this scene, Mickey (Woody Allen) comes to his physician with a variety of vague complaints, and then returns to work.

1  What are the symptoms of generalized anxiety disorder (GAD) as revealed by Micky?
2  How does GAD differ from other anxiety disorders? How much overlap is there between GAD and other mental disorders, including somatization?
3  What are the most effective ways to reassure an overly anxious patient?
4  What are successful pharmacologic and non-pharmacologic approaches to the treatment of patients with GAD?

## Obsessive-compulsive disorder

◆ *As Good as it Gets* (Jack Nicholson, Helen Hunt). This is an award-winning movie about Melvin Udall (Jack Nicholson), a novelist, and his relationship with Carol Connelly (Helen Hunt), a kind-hearted waitress.

a (0:40:34–0:44:03). In this succession of scenes Melvin is having a 'bad' day. This clip begins with him barging into his therapist's office and ends with him being evicted from a restaurant.

1 What symptoms of obsessive-compulsive disorder (OCD) does Melvin demonstrate in these scenes?
2 What are the most common presentations of OCD in medical practice? Why is it relatively easy to miss?
3 What are the most effective pharmacologic and non-pharmacologic approaches to OCD?
4 Distinguish between OCD and obsessive-compulsive personality disorder (OCPD).


## Agoraphobia

◆ *Copycat* (Sigourney Weaver, Holly Hunter, Dermot Mulroney). Dr Helen Hudson (Sigourney Weaver), an authority on serial killers, nearly becomes a victim herself. As a result of being attacked, she develops agoraphobia. A year after her attack she reluctantly agrees to help Inspectors Monaghan (Holly Hunter) and Getz (Dermot Mulroney) find a serial killer in San Francisco.

a. (0:18:47–0:20:00). Dr Hudson is seen trying to retrieve her newspaper, which is beyond her grasp. She tries to reach it with a broom, but each effort forces her to extend herself further and further outside her door. She begins to panic and starts to recite the names of the presidents to distract herself. Finally, as the hallway seems to grow, she successfully lunges for the paper.

1 In this scene, what role does Dr Hudson's repetitious behavior serve?

b. (0:27:30–0:28:45). Inspectors Monaghan and Getz arrive at Dr Hudson's apartment. When they bring out the crime-scene photos Dr Hudson begins to hyperventilate, and she calls for her houseman. He arrives with a paper bag and assures the officers that paramedics are not needed. He explains that Dr Hudson is having a panic attack and that she will be fine in half an hour. He further states that she has not been outside her house for a year and that she suffers from agoraphobia.

1 How do families, friends and associates respond to individuals who experience panic attacks?
2 What efforts do patients make to 'self-treat' symptoms of panic?

c (1:02:25–1:04:10). Dr Hudson discovers that the police officer who is guarding her is not at his post and that her phone lines are dead. She sees someone outside her apartment. She begins to hyperventilate as she crawls along the walls outside her apartment in a hand-over-hand motion. Everything begins to spin around her. She progresses only a few feet before she turns and runs back into her apartment, despite the potential danger that awaits her there.

1 Have you ever known or treated someone with agoraphobia?
2 How best can you encourage agoraphobics to overcome their fears for long enough to get to your office?
3 What are successful treatment strategies for agoraphobia?

## Somatoform disorder

### Somatization disorder

◆ *Hannah and Her Sisters* (Woody Allen, Mia Farrow). See earlier section on generalized anxiety disorder for movie description.

a (0:14:02–0:18:19). In this scene, Mickey (Woody Allen) comes to his physician with a variety of vague complaints, and then returns to work.

1 What symptoms of somatization disorder are demonstrated by Micky?
2 Differentiate between syndromal and sub-syndromal presentations of somatization disorder.
3 How effectively does the first doctor in this scene alleviate Micky's anxiety? What are some positive and negative aspects of his approach? Compare this doctor with the second doctor, who gives Micky a telephone consultation.
4 Does somatization disorder run in families? If so, why?
5 Distinguish somatization disorder from hypochondriasis.
6 What are effective primary care approaches to the somaticizing patient?
7 What are common physician reactions to somaticizers?

### Conversion disorder

◆ *Hollywood Ending* (Woody Allen, Tea Leoni). Val Waxman (Woody Allen) is a movie director whose ex-wife (Tea Leoni) chooses him to shoot a new movie in an effort to help rejuvenate his career. This reversal of fortune provokes performance anxiety and insecurity in Waxman, emotions that find expression in psychosomatic blindness illustrative of conversion disorder.

a (0:40:14–0:44:30). Waxman calls his agent in a crisis – he has fallen asleep on his couch and awoken blind. A series of tests performed by medical experts determines the lack of organic etiology. A psychotherapist diagnoses Waxman's blindness as a classic case of psychosomatic illness.

1 Of what psychiatric diagnosis is this clip illustrative?
2 What is the theoretical understanding of conversion disorder?
3 How do you explain *unexplainable* symptoms to a patient?
4 How do you reassure a patient (and their family) who is experiencing dramatic life-altering, unexplained symptoms?
5 If Waxman was your medical patient, how would you proceed? If you were to make a referral to a psychotherapist, how would you proceed? How successful do you believe such a referral would be?

## References

1. Sharp L, Lipsky M. Screening for depression across the lifespan: a review of measures for use in primary care settings. *Am Fam Physician* 2002; **66**: 1001–8.
2. Manderscheid RW, Rae DS, Narrow WE *et al.* Congruence of service utilization estimates from the epidemiological catchment area project and other sources. *Arch Gen Psychiatry* 1993; **50**: 108–14.
3. Staab JP, Datto CJ, Weinrieb RM *et al.* Detection and diagnosis of psychiatric disorders in primary medical care settings. *Med Clin North Am* 2001; **85**: 579–96.
4. Gerber PD, Barret JE, Barrett JA. Recognition of depression by internists in primary care: a comparison of internist and 'gold standard' psychiatric assessments. *J Gen Intern Med* 1989; **4**: 7–13.

# Chapter 12

# Chemical dependency

*Matthew Alexander and Patricia Lenahan*

Chemical dependency is one of the most important, challenging and ultimately rewarding problems treated by healthcare providers. The list of substances to which patients may be addicted is long – nicotine, alcohol, prescription drugs and illicit drugs which themselves are often changing to mirror the tastes of young abusers. Chemical dependency is important because of the staggering social cost of addiction, the comorbidity between chemical dependence and such medical conditions as chronic pain, depression/anxiety, cancer, developmental delay (for newborn infants of addicts), chronic obstructive pulmonary disease (COPD) and heart disease, and the disproportionate rates at which chemically dependent patients present as outpatients and inpatients.

Chemical dependency is a challenging problem for healthcare professionals because of a variety of factors. Due to the sheer power of physical and emotional addiction and the shame associated with it, chemically dependent patients are usually guarded about their addiction and highly resistant to habit change. Consequently, healthcare providers in busy practices can easily miss the diagnosis[1] or have unconscious reasons to avoid making the diagnosis. In addition, there are high rates of relapse and multiple hidden 'victims,' enablers and co-addicts within the family.

However, chemical dependency is also a very rewarding problem to treat in clinical practice. There are few individuals as grateful to providers for helping to fight their illness as former addicts in recovery! Luckily for educators, there is a wealth of films from which to choose that are useful in helping learners to understand, diagnose and treat chemical dependency.

## Alcoholism

◆ *When a Man Loves a Woman* (Andy Garcia, Meg Ryan). This movie is a treasure trove for teaching about alcoholism and its impact on the family. Alice (Meg Ryan) and Michael (Andy Garcia) are married with two daughters. Alice struggles with alcoholism and Michael struggles to be a supportive husband and father.

a (0:30:40–0:35:57). In this scene, Alice comes home intoxicated. After dismissing the babysitter, she proceeds to chase aspirin with vodka, hit her daughter and fall through the shower glass, unconscious.

1  What aspects of alcoholism are revealed in this clip?
2  How might Alice present to her primary care provider? What are common clinical clues to the presence of alcoholism?

3  What are the best ways to diagnose and confront alcoholics in your practice?
4  What resources for alcoholics are available in your community?
5  What is the impact of alcoholism on children? What treatment options are available for children of alcoholics? What are the characteristics of adult children of alcoholics?
6  How successful have you been in identifying and treating chemically dependent patients in your practice? Have you known personally any individuals struggling with addiction?

b  (0:35:58–0:39:11). Alice is taken to the hospital after her fall. In this clip, Michael is at her bedside as they discuss her drinking history.

1  What aspects of alcoholism are revealed in this scene?
2  What aspects of codependency are revealed in this scene?
3  How might codependents present in clinical practice?
4  What treatment options are available for codependents?
5  Are healthcare professionals codependent? When does codependency become a problem for the healthcare professional?

◆  *Drunks* (Richard Lewis, Faye Dunaway, Dianne Wiest). This film provides an in-depth look at the 12-step recovery process as it follows an ethnically and socially diverse group of individuals who share their stories during an AA meeting.

a  (0:07:46–0:13:57). In this clip, Jim (Richard Lewis) is called upon to share his story at an AA meeting. He describes his childhood with an alcoholic father and his own experimentation/use of alcohol as a preteen and during high school. When alcohol no longer got him high, he switched to heroin. In this scene, he talks about quitting and how he ended up at AA.

1  What factors have contributed to this individual's substance abuse? How does hearing Jim's history affect your empathy toward his drinking and heroin use? Do you think knowing a patient's psychological history would impact attitudes in the emergency room or other health centers?
2  What role does denial play in Jim's description of his problem?
3  What factors are most predictive of successful cessation and recovery?
4  What factors are likely to trigger a relapse?
5  How illustrative of AA is this scene? What is your understanding of the hows and whys of 12-step programs such as AA?
6  Is AA sufficient for substance abuse treatment? Discuss the role of individual therapy.

## Cocaine addiction

◆  *Blow* (Johnny Depp, Penelope Cruz, Ray Liotta, Paul Reubens, Franka Potente, Jordi Molla). This powerful film tells the true story of George Jung (Johnny Depp), who was the largest importer of Colombian cocaine to the USA in the 1970s and 1980s.

a  (0:31:47–0:37:06). George tells how he skipped bail to take care of his girlfriend, Barbara (Franka Potente). He is now a fugitive and is visiting his parents. His mother contacts the police. They arrive and take George away.

1   What are the different ways in which parents respond to their children's drug use and criminal activities?
2   Is there a connection between parental use of chemicals and children's use of chemicals?
3   How would you advise a parent to deal with a child (minor or adult) who is making bad choices in their life?

b   (0:53:09–0:54:57). George and his drug-dealing partners are at a gathering and measure the purity of the cocaine.

1   How do you understand the continuing demand for cocaine in this country?
2   How do you assess for cocaine use and abuse in your outpatient practice?
3   What are the physical dangers associated with cocaine use?
4   What are the different means of ingesting cocaine? What are the dangers associated with each method? What is the addictive potential of each method? How does cocaine addiction compare with other types of chemical addiction?
5   What treatment programs are available locally for patients with cocaine addiction?

c   (1:17:10–1:23:42). George's partner, Diego (Jordi Molla), makes a deal without him. George confronts his former partner, who is on a cocaine binge, and physically assaults him. Later, George is bingeing before his daughter is born. At the delivery, he collapses and is thought to have had a heart attack.

1   What is the association between chronic cocaine use and mood swings?
2   What is the association between chronic drug use and paranoia, delusions and violence?
3   What is the best treatment for individuals who need to be detoxified?
4   How effective is the physician who gives advice to George in the hospital?
5   What barriers does the drug-addicted individual face when they attempt sobriety? What are the best indicators of successful drug recovery?

d   (1:34:16–1:35:48). George's wife is snorting cocaine in the car and yells at him. She asks him why he has not touched her for so long. The car swerves and they are pulled over by the police. George's wife tells the police that he is a fugitive drug dealer.

1   What is the association between drug use and domestic violence?

# Heroin addiction

◆ *Permanent Midnight* (Ben Stiller, Elizabeth Hurley). This is a true story about a successful television writer who becomes addicted to heroin and other drugs before eventually recovering.

a   (0:28:15–0:33:49). We see a typical day for Jerry (Ben Stiller), beginning with him shooting heroin, then showing up late at work, leaving to get his next fix and finally lying to his wife about why he is late for their dinner appointment.

1   What stereotypes of heroin abuse does this scene illustrate? What stereotypes does it dispel?

2 Has Jerry hit bottom yet? What do you predict will happen to him if he does not get help?

3 Why do addicts lie to those to whom they are closest?

4 Have you ever known or treated heroin addicts? If so, what was your experience like?

b (0:45:00–0:46:56). Jerry is offered a new job as a writer for a television show. It provides the impetus for him to get a medical evaluation for methadone maintenance.

1 Comment on the physician's interviewing style. Have you ever felt this discouraged about abusers?

2 How often do addicts relapse before they either die or become sober?

c (0:59:56–1:09:33). This is a disturbing scene in which Jerry takes his baby on an aborted drug buy. The scene illustrates the complete and utter desperation of the addict and what 'bottom' truly looks like.

1 What feelings does this scene evoke in you?

2 Have you known patients who have put children or other loved ones in jeopardy because of their addiction? What has been your reaction to this? How does one best handle negative emotions towards patients?

## Marijuana abuse

◆ *Blow* (Johnny Depp, Penelope Cruz, Ray Liotta, Paul Reubens). See earlier section on cocaine addiction for movie description.

a. (0:07:12–0:08:58, 0:13:26–0:15:08). In these scenes, George and his friend Tuna move to California and become intimately acquainted with a circle of friends who routinely use marijuana.

1 How do you screen for marijuana use in clinical practice?

2 What are the positive experiences associated with marijuana use as highlighted by these movie clips? Why is it important to acknowledge the positive impact of chemicals if you are trying to motivate patients to stop or cut down on their usage?

3 What are the dangers associated with marijuana abuse? When does its use become a problem?

4 Do you believe that marijuana is a gateway drug? If so, why? If not, why not?

5 What are the unique challenges associated with chemical dependency treatment of patients with a history of marijuana abuse?

6 Distinguish between chemical non-use, use, abuse, addiction and dependence.

## Teenage drug abuse

◆ *Kids* (Leo Kirkpatrick, Justin Pierce, Chloe Sevigny). This is a very powerful and disturbing film that looks at a day in the lives of several urban teenagers who are experimenting with drugs and sex. It provides a vivid insight into the thought processes of teenagers, their feelings of invincibility and the fallacy of their cognitions. This film is raw and real – it is not a film for the faint-hearted.

a (0:11:36–013:50). A group of adolescent boys are sitting around smoking joints and inhaling nitrous oxide through balloons. They quickly become 'high' from the marijuana and inhalant use.

1  What is the prevalence of inhalant use among adolescents?
2  What effects does inhalant use have on overall health?
3  The boys depicted here also use marijuana and alcohol. What is the prevalence of adolescent polydrug abuse?
4  What types of interventions are helpful with adolescent drug abusers?
5  What is the role of the family doctor in prevention of drug abuse?


## Prescription drug abuse

◆ *Requiem for a Dream* (Ellen Burstyn, Jennifer Connally). This is a film about Sara (Ellen Burstyn), a lonely widowed mother, and her son, his girlfriend and his best friend. They all struggle with addictive issues.

a (0:28:49–0:29:29). In this clearly exaggerated scene, Sara goes to see a physician who prescribes her weight-loss drugs even though he has had very little previous contact with her. Sadly, she rapidly becomes profoundly addicted to these drugs.

1  Why is this scene a relevant stereotype of physicians?
2  How *does* a physician walk the thin line between being sensitive to patients' needs for psychoactive prescription drugs while also being alert to the addictive potential of these drugs?
3  What are some of the most dangerous prescribed drugs you have given to patients? How have you safeguarded yourself against becoming an unwitting enabler for a patient's addiction?

b (0:35:04–0:36:33). In this scene, which should be shown immediately after the one previously cited, we see the profound and destructive impact of the stimulants prescribed by Sara's physician.


## Geriatric substance abuse

◆ *A Thousand Acres* (Jason Robards, Jessica Lange, Michele Pfeiffer, Jennifer Jason Leigh). Based on a Pulitzer-prize-winning book of the same name, *A Thousand Acres* is a portrait of the Cook family. Like Shakespeare's King Lear, family patriarch Larry Cook (Jason Robards) is facing his own mortality and brings his three daughters together to discuss forming a corporation to divide the family farm. When his lawyer daughter (Jennifer Jason Leigh) expresses doubt about this plan, Larry becomes enraged. Viewers are then given an insight into the family and their secrets.

a (0:27:00–0:28:58). Rose (Michele Pfeiffer) and Ginny (Jessica Lange) are talking about their father. Rose asks Ginny what she really thinks of him. Ginny says that he drinks and probably has done so for as long as they have known him, but that 'Mama never told us what to think about Daddy.'

b (0:33:55–0:35:42). Rose receives a call from the hospital. Her father is in the ER following an alcohol-related accident. On the way home from the hospital, Ginny begins questioning him, asking her father if he has the pills that the nurse gave him. She appears angry and threatens to take away his truck. She warns him that he should not be drinking and driving.

1 What are some considerations for assessing substance abuse in older adults?
2 When assessing possible substance abuse in the elderly, differential diagnosis is essential because alcohol abuse can mimic other conditions. Identify three such disorders that might be uncovered through differential diagnosis.
3 Why are older adults at risk for alcohol/drug problems?
4 What is the prognosis for an individual like Larry who has been drinking all his life and who has minimal family support?

## Reference

1.  Fleming MF. Strategies to increase alcohol screening in health care settings. *Alcohol Health Res World* 1997; **21**: 340–7.

# Chapter 13

# Family violence

Colleen Fogarty, Patricia Lenahan, Matthew Alexander, Amy Ellwood, Alexandra Duke and Layne Prest

Violence affects men, women and children, although women bear the brunt of the medical and mental health sequelae. The Centers for Disease Control (CDC), the World Health Organization (WHO) and the United Nations identify violence against women as a major public health issue.[1–4] Victims of violence often seek medical care long after their physical injuries have healed. Psychological problems, somatic complaints, revictimization and post-traumatic stress disorders (PTSD) are among the many problems that victims of violence continue to experience.[5–9]

Children who live in homes where violence occurs are also at risk for physical, emotional, sexual and psychological abuse.[10,11] As adults, they are likely to repeat the pattern of abuse, become victims themselves and/or develop chronic health problems. In addition the majority of child abductions and child homicides are committed by parents or parental figures.

Victims of intimate partner violence and their children may also be exposed to violence directed towards their pets. Abuse of companion animals is highly correlated with the development of child abuse and other forms of violence. Often the abuse of companion animals may serve as a precursor to the onset of violence in the home.

Family physicians are in an ideal position to assess, diagnose and treat the victims of intimate partner violence through identification and screening of all patients. Effective assessment and intervention are most likely when physicians regularly consider family abuse as a possible core problem, conduct routine screening and provide continuity of care. Yet many physicians have little training in violence-related issues and are hesitant to ask the all-important questions that are needed to assess patients and their personal relationships.[12,13]

Many of the following scenes depict graphic violence that may be difficult to view. These scenes may also trigger emotional reactions in those who have experienced some form of violence in their own lives or who suffer from 'compassion fatigue.'

## Child abuse

◆ *Radio Flyer* (Lorraine Bracco, John Heard, Ben Johnson, Adam Baldwin, Elijah Wood, Joseph Mazzello). This movie is narrated in part by Tom Hanks, who as an adult recalls his childhood. *Radio Flyer* illustrates the malevolent nature of child physical abuse in a stepfamily, and the children's attempt to protect their mother and cope through fantasies and escapism.

a (0:33:41–0:36:00). The 'King' (Adam Baldwin) comes home and starts drinking. He is physically and emotionally abusive to the children. He sends Mike (Elijah Wood), the older of the two boys, to bed and then physically abuses Bobbie (Joseph Mazzello), who cannot lie on his back afterwards.

b (0:50:25–0:53:44). The boys arrive home to find all of their toys and clothes thrown on the lawn. Mike says to Bobbie that they need to clean it up before their mom sees it. Boys in the neighborhood are bullying Mike and Bobbie. The sheriff drives by, breaks up the fight and asks them if they need any help. He gives the boys his card and tells them to call him if they need anything.

c (01:06:24–01:07:36). Bobbie is in a hospital bed lying down. His eyes are black and his mother promises that this will never happen again. She tells him that his stepfather is in jail. Bobbie wants to talk with Mike alone, so their mother leaves the bedside.

d (1:11:52–1:14:24). ''The King' arrives at the house with flowers for his wife and gifts for the boys. He obtained early release from jail to attend his mother's funeral. He begs for forgiveness from his wife, tells her that it will never happen again, that he will stop drinking and that he loves her. The children recall their mother saying that he was never coming back. However, they realize that she still needs him and is faced with one of the hardest decisions she has ever had to make.

1 Is child abuse more or less common in stepfamilies? Why?
2 What can parents do to become more aware of possible sexual, physical or emotional abuse occurring in their own home?
3 What are some of the challenges faced by stepfamilies as they attempt to build family cohesion?
4 Why did the mother in this clip take her abusive husband back? What impact do you think this had on her children?
5 As a healthcare professional, what steps can you take to prevent and/or identify child abuse?
6 What are the potential long-term physical and emotional sequelae of childhood exposure to violence?
7 What is the role of law enforcement in identifying and/or preventing child abuse and intimate partner violence?

## Emotional and physical abuse

◆ *Prince of Tides* (Barbra Streisand, Nick Nolte, Blythe Danner, Melinda Dillon, Kate Nelligan). This film, based on a novel by Pat Conroy, deals with family sequelae of domestic violence. Set in coastal South Carolina and New York City, it chronicles the life of Tom Wingo (Nick Nolte), the narrator and main character, as he travels to New York to 'be the memory' for his mentally troubled sister, Savannah (Melinda Dillon), who has made another suicide attempt.

The family systems dynamics, as well as the depiction of individual responses to childhood violence, make this movie an important teaching resource. Through a series of flashbacks, Tom recounts to his psychiatrist violence by his father towards his mother, the resistance strategies of his mother and the psychological abuse that she in turn inflicted on her children.

a (0:23:24–0:24:25). This is a dinner-table scene in the Wingo household. It is a flashback scene initiated by Tom as he cooks a shrimp meal for himself while in New York. Lila Wingo (Kate Nelligan), Tom's mother, has prepared Shrimp Newburgh for dinner, and Henry Wingo (Brad Sullivan) starts to complain and insult his wife. Tom, the younger son, chimes in, 'I think it's pretty good.' Henry responds to his son's comment by saying 'Who asked you?', and goes on to verbally abuse Tom, 'You ain't going to cry, are you?' Then he turns to Savannah and says 'Go get this little girl one of your dresses.'

1   What stage of the cycle of violence does this scene demonstrate?
2   What is the impact on the children?
3   How might the verbal abuse that Tom receives from his father affect his emotional development?

## Childhood sexual abuse and incest

◆ *The Color Purple* (Danny Glover, Whoopi Goldberg, Oprah Winfrey). This film adaptation of the novel by Alice Walker tells the story of the maturation of Celia (Whoopi Goldberg), an African-American woman who is molested and has two children by her father.

a (0:03:15–0:06:35). In this scene, Celia is giving birth to a baby daughter. Her father, also the baby's father, is looming in the distance. He takes the newborn baby out of Celia's arms, warning her not to tell her mother so as not to 'break her heart.' In the next scene, Celia is walking behind her mother's hearse, trying to make sense of her life.

1   What is the prevalence of incest in our society? What is its prevalence in other societies?
2   What is the impact of incest on victims and families?
3   What are the best treatment strategies for incest survivors?

## Impact of childhood sexual abuse on adult functioning

◆ *Bliss* (Craig Sheffer, Sheryl Lee, Terence Stamp, Spalding Gray). This movie focuses on the relationship issues of a newly married couple. Maria (Sheryl Lee) has a history of obsessive-compulsive disorder and suicidal ideation. She has seen four therapists in seven years, and has also been described as having bipolar disorder. Maria admits to her husband, Joseph (Craig Sheffer), that she is anorgasmic, which sends the couple on a course of self-discovery that leads to Maria's memories of being sexually molested as a child. With the help of her therapist, Alfred (Spalding Gray), and her sex therapist, Balthazar (Terence Stamp), the couple begin to confront the effects of the abuse on their marriage.

a (1:16:35–1:17:14). This brief clip shows Maria at a support group meeting. She introduces herself as a survivor of child sexual abuse and incest. As she is talking, viewers see her telling her mother about the abuse. The scene shifts to Maria at home, with Joseph complaining about her taking five showers. Maria says that she sees *him*, her father, when they are making love. She tells Joseph that she is going crazy and wants to separate from him.

1 What is the therapeutic value of identifying oneself as a survivor of child sexual abuse?
2 What are the long-term effects of childhood sexual abuse?
3 How does post-traumatic stress disorder manifest itself when the victimization has not been acknowledged?

b (1:26:30–1:31:45). Joseph receives a call from Maria's therapist, Alfred, asking him to attend a session. Maria volunteers to talk about the memories of her childhood sexual abuse first. Joseph listens to his wife's painful history and then talks to the therapist about Maria.

1 What are the effects of childhood sexual abuse on adult relationships?
2 How would you counsel the partner of an incest survivor regarding intimacy and trust issues?

## The cycle of violence and physical abuse

◆ *Sleeping with the Enemy* (Julia Roberts, Patrick Bergin, Kevin Anderson). Julia Roberts portrays Laura, who is married to Martin Burney (Patrick Bergin), a compulsive, controlling and violent man. Laura fakes her own death as the only way she has of leaving the marriage and beginning a new life in the Midwest.

a (0:05:51–0:12:56). In this series of scenes, the nature of the relationship between Martin and Laura is elucidated and an episode of intimate partner violence is enacted when Martin suspects Laura of flirting with a physician neighbor. After he leaves, Laura struggles to get to her feet.

1 What elements of domestic violence does this clip illustrate?
2 What is the relationship between domestic violence and excessive need for control?
3 What causes a woman to stay in a violent relationship? What are the dangers when she attempts to leave?
4 Discuss the cycle of violence as illustrated in this clip.
5 What is the best way to screen for intimate partner violence in practice?
6 What resources are available in your community for victims of intimate partner violence?

◆ *Enough* (Jennifer Lopez, Bill Campbell, Juliette Lewis, Noah Wylie). Slim (Jennifer Lopez), a small-town waitress, marries a man (Bill Campbell) who uses both his financial power and his physical strength to control her. When Slim confronts her husband about the fact that he is having an affair, he slaps her for the first time. Slim utilizes the support of her friends to try to escape from her husband, while experiencing the consequences of her husband's rage and need to control.

a (0:29:25–0:35:54). Slim attempts to leave her husband and has arranged for her friends to pick her up in the middle of the night. Her husband awakens and starts to beat her in front of their sleeping child. When her friends break into the house, her husband threatens them with a gun, but he lets them leave when his daughter sees her father with the gun.

1   What are the risks for women who attempt to leave abusive situations?
2   What could Slim have done differently to protect herself and her daughter when leaving the abusive relationship?
3   What is the role of law enforcement in domestic violence situations?
4   Why are victims hesitant to contact the police?

◆ *What's Love Got To Do With It?* (Laurence Fishburne, Angela Bassett). This movie is a dramatic portrayal of the relationship between Ike (Laurence Fishburne) and Tina Turner (Angela Bassett). It is a realistic and gripping depiction of the escalation of control, intimidation and multi-level violence in an intimate relationship. The story also illuminates the many barriers that deter women from leaving an abusive relationship, but is optimistic in that it shows how one woman was able to leave successfully. An important part of the movie is the lyrics of songs written by Ike and performed by Tina. The lyrics chronicle the evolution of their relationship, but also provide a commentary on the socially and culturally embedded messages that enable the abuse of power to be disguised by intimacy and confused with love.

a   (0:38:50–0:43:17). At this point in the film, Annie Mae is becoming 'Tina Turner.' She has a baby with Ike and they go to Mexico to get married. However, the shine is starting to wear off as he cajoles and manipulates her despite her protestations. She seems to be ignorant of the warning bells in her own mind and sings 'Things are gonna work out fine.'

1   What are the signs of increasing power and control tactics being used by Ike?
2   Discuss the '8 Fs' which represent the barriers to women leaving abusive relationships (fear, family, feelings, finances, faith, forgiveness, fatigue and fantasy). How are these manifested in this relationship?
3   What are the risks of physical violence during pregnancy?
4   What areas of family/marital relationships do you assess with pregnant patients?

# Delusional stalking

◆ *One Hour Photo* (Robin Williams, Dylan Smith, Connie Nielsen, Michael Vartan). In a brilliant portrayal, Robin Williams plays Sy Parrish, a one-hour photo technician who has dutifully developed photos for the Yorkin family since their son was small. A lonely, isolated bachelor, Parrish becomes increasingly delusional about his relationship with the family.

a   (0:11:14–0:19:30). In this series of scenes, we witness Sy falsely stating to a waitress that the Yorkins' son (Dylan Smith) is his nephew, gain insight into the conflicts within the Yorkin family and confront the full range of Sy's obsession with the Yorkin family.

1   How would you diagnose Sy?
2   How did you feel when the full extent of Sy's obsession with the Yorkin family

was revealed? How do you believe victims feel when they become aware that someone is obsessed with them and may in fact be stalking them?

3  What is the relationship between obsessive-compulsive disorder, obsessive-compulsive personality disorder and stalking?

b (0:28:54–0:32:30). In this powerful scene we see Sy watch the Yorkin home from his car and then break in while the family is out. Sy is seen walking through the rooms, using the toilet, sitting in the living room and then being greeted by the family when they return as if he were a beloved uncle. We find out that his entry into the home is a fantasy.

1  Have you ever worked with delusional patients? How do you understand the phenomenon of having delusions?
2  What are the most effective treatments for delusional disorders?
3  What is the link between delusions and stalking?
4  How do you define stalking? Have you or has anyone you know ever been stalked? What are the emotional effects of being stalked?
5  What is the association between social immaturity/isolation and stalking?
6  What is the best way to treat individuals in your practice who are stalkers or who are being stalked?
7  How does delusional stalking differ from the stalking that occurs in intimate partner relationships? What are the dynamics in intimate partner violence-related stalking?

## Child witnesses to intimate partner violence

◆ *Enough* (Jennifer Lopez, Noah Wylie). See earlier section on the cycle of violence and physical abuse for movie description.

a (0:55:28–0:56:10). Slim believes that her daughter will be cheered up if she talks with her father. During the telephone call, Slim's daughter hears her father swearing and threatening her mother on the phone. He realizes that he is not talking to Slim and that his daughter has heard what he said. He apologizes and she quietly ends the phone call.

b (1:08:00–1:09:10). Slim's husband finds Slim and their daughter. He tells Slim that he wants her back. He threatens her and says that if he cannot have her then no one will. He begins hitting Slim while their daughter tries to pull him off. During the process, the little girl is shoved and thrown to the ground.

1  What is the impact of domestic violence on children?
2  What are some of the typical behavioral and emotional consequences of domestic violence for children?
3  What interventions would be helpful for a child who is exposed to domestic violence?

◆ *What's Love Got To Do With It?* (Laurence Fishburne, Angela Bassett). See earlier section on the cycle of violence and physical abuse for movie description.

a (0:54:15–0:58:28). This scene is a fairly graphic portrayal of the emotional and physical violence in the relationship between Ike and Tina Turner. It also portrays the impact that violence has on their children, and the role of their community of friends and associates. Despite being beaten in front of her friends and children, Tina makes excuses for her husband's behavior.

1 How can a woman and her abusive partner ignore or be oblivious to the effects that intimate partner violence has on their children?
2 What is the role of extended family, friends and community in intervening in domestic disputes?
3 At what stage of readiness for change is Tina at this point in the movie (in contrast to earlier scenes)?
4 What does this scene suggest about the natural history of intimate partner violence and the cycle of violence?

## Impact of substance abuse on intimate partner violence and childhood exposure to trauma

◆ *Smoke Signals* (Adam Beach, Evan Adams). This is the story of two young American Indians from the Coeur D'Alene tribe who leave the reservation to bring home the ashes of one of their fathers.

a (0:25:22–0:31:06). The parents of Victor (Adam Beach) are seen at a party. Both of them have been drinking. The scene shifts to the parents in bed, still wearing their clothes and Victor outside, smashing beer bottles. His mother wakes up and sees what her son is doing. She wakes her husband and says that they have to stop drinking. A fight erupts in which Victor's father slaps his mother, pushing her to the ground. She tells him to get out. Victor is seen running after his father.

1 What role does alcohol or drug use play in violence?
2 How did Victor's behavior contribute to his mother's awareness of the impact of parental alcohol use on her son?
3 What are the emotional consequences for children who are exposed to both violence and alcohol/drugs?

b (0:32:20–0:33:30). Victor's mother is hugging him and telling him that his father has gone. Victor's friend Thomas comes over and says that he has heard that Victor's father has left. He asks Victor if his dad left because he hates him. Victor beats up Thomas.

1 What factors contributed to this violence?
2 What is the impact of parental violence on children's behavior?
3 What interventions are needed to prevent Victor from repeating his father's behavior in adult relationships with intimate partners?

c (1:03:13–1:04:49). Thomas and Victor are driving back to the reservation. Thomas is telling stories about Victor's father and how kind he was. Victor becomes agitated and tells Thomas that he does not know anything about his father, and says he was a drunk who beat both his mother and him.

1 How do public perceptions of batterers differ from private realities?
2 How do perpetrators of violence hide their abusive nature from others?

3 How does this disconnection between public perception and private reality contribute to self-doubt and demoralization in victims?

## Family violence and homicide

◆ *In the Bedroom* (Sissy Spacek, Tom Wilkinson, Nick Stahl, Marisa Tomei). This movie addresses the pervasive nature of domestic violence in our society and clearly shows how many victims are created by family violence. Music director Ruth Fowler (Sissy Spacek) and her family physician husband, Matt Fowler (Tom Wilkinson), attempt to cope with the loss of their only son, Frank (Nick Stahl), who was murdered by his girlfriend Natalie's (Marisa Tomei) abusive and violent estranged husband, Richard. While the overwhelming theme of this film focuses on family relationships and coping with loss, it also offers a vivid exposure to domestic violence, its impact on children and the tragic consequences that may occur when interventions are lacking.

a (0:07:37–00:39:21). In this scene, Frank is at Natalie's home when her explosive ex-husband, Richard, shows up. Her two sons are terrified as she tries to get them to hide in the bedroom. Natalie's ex-husband trashes her house, yells and threatens Frank, and then leaves the house and returns with a gun. Richard shoots Frank in the head as Natalie comes running down the stairs.

1 Could this senseless act of violence have been prevented?
2 What effect will Richard's actions have on his two young sons?
3 Is it possible to reason with a man in a rage similar to Richard, Natalie's estranged husband?

b (1:42:00–1:55:30). In these scenes Dr Matt Fowler kidnaps, shoots and kills Richard, the man who killed his son.

1 What causes this respectable physician to plan the murder of his son's killer?
2 Is Dr Fowler's premeditated murder of his son's killer any different to the rage-induced murder of his son? Do you feel that Dr Fowler's actions were justified?
3 What could have been done to prevent this violence?

## Sexual assault

Sexual assault is the fastest-growing violent crime in the USA. When survivors of rape testify in court, they are often revictimized when they are cross-examined by defense attorneys. Healthcare providers must understand the horrific nature of sexual assault, the context in which it occurs and the emotional impact of acts forced upon the victim in order to provide appropriate care.

◆ *The Accused* (Jodie Foster, Kelly McGillis). This movie is the story of Sarah Tobias (Jodie Foster), a woman who was gang raped, and the prosecutor (Kelly McGillis) who helps her to find justice.

a (0:2:30–0:07:00). Sarah Tobias flees the rape scene and goes to the emergency room where the rape protocol is depicted.

b (1:04:00–1:09:20). Sarah is testifying about what happened that night. We see what occurred in the game room at the back of the bar. Sarah is raped on a pinball machine while other men cheer the perpetrator and take turns assaulting her. A female waitress looks on in a conspiracy of silence.

1  Gang rape is most common among adolescents and college students. Why might this be so?
2  What are the immediate and long-term psychological consequences of rape?
3  What can physicians do during the immediate care of rape survivors to empower them?

## Companion animal abuse

◆ *Radio Flyer* (Lorraine Bracco, John Heard, Ben Johnson, Adam Baldwin, Elijah Wood, Joseph Mazzello). See earlier section on child abuse for movie description.

a (1:24:31–1:28:15). The two brothers, Bobbie and Mike, are eating at school when both complain about having upset stomachs. Using a split-screen approach, the director shows the two boys running home while their stepfather simultaneously arrives home, has a beer and hears the family dog, Shane, barking. Bobbie and Mike come home and start calling for Shane. Seeing blood on the sliding glass door, they begin a search for their dog. Shane appears to be dead at first, but he then whimpers while both boys hold him. Bobbie and Mike decide that it is time for Bobbie (who has previously been physically abused by the stepfather), Shane and Sampson (the family tortoise) to leave.

1  What types of things are learned by children who witness the abuse of companion animals?
2  What is the impact on attachment when children witness abuse or the murder of a pet?
3  What types of behavior might be seen in a child whose beloved pet has been killed by an abusive family member?
4  If a patient reported that their pet had been injured by an abusive partner, would it increase your index of suspicion for other types of abuse?

## *References*

1.  Tjaden P, Thoennes N. Prevalence and consequences of male-to-female and female-to-male partner violence as measured by the National Violence Against Women Survey. *Violence Against Women* 2000; **6**: 142–61.
2.  Tjaden P, Thoennes N. *Full Report of the Prevalence, Incidence and Consequences of Violence Against Women.* Washington, DC: US Department of Justice, 2000.
3.  Auchter B, Campbell J, Ganley A. *Intimate Partner Surveillance: uniform definitions and recommended data elements, verson 1.0.* Atlanta GA: National Center for Injury Prevention and Control, Centers for Disease Control and Prevention, 1999.
4.  Leawood KS. *Family Violence.* Leawood KA: American Academy of Family Physicians, 2000; www.aafp.org/x7132.xml
5.  Ulrich YC, Cain K, Sugg NK. Medical care utilization patterns in women with diagnosed domestic violence. *Am J Prev Med* 2003; **24**: 9–15.
6.  Acierno R, Resnick HS, Kilpatrick DG. Health impact of interpersonal violence: prevalence rates, case identification and risk factors for sexual assault, physical assault and domestic violence in men and women. *Behav Med* 1997; **23**: 53–64.

7. Coker AL, Smith PH, Bethea L. Physical health consequences of physical and psychological intimate partner violence. *Arch Fam Med* 2000; **9**: 451–7.

8. Coker AL, Davis AE, Arias I. Physical and mental health effects of intimate partner violence for men and women. *Am J Prev Med* 2002; **23**: 260–8.

9. McCauley J, Kern DE, Kolodner K. Relation of low-severity violence to women's health. *J Gen Intern Med* 1998; **13**: 687–91.

10. McCauley J, Kern DE, Kolodner K. Clinical characteristics of women with a history of childhood abuse: unhealed wounds. *JAMA* 1997; **277**: 1362–8.

11. McCloskey LA, Figueredo AJ, Koss MP. The effects of systemic family violence on children's mental health. *Child Dev* 1995; **66**: 1239–61.

12. Sugg NK, Inui T. Primary care physician's response to domestic violence: opening Pandora's box. *JAMA* 1992; **267**: 3157–60.

13. Rodriguez MA, Bauer HM, McLoughlin E. Screening and intervention for intimate partner abuse: practices and attitudes of primary care physicians. *JAMA* 1999; **282**: 468–74.

Chapter 14

# Schizophrenia and bipolar disorders

*Anna Pavlov*

The assessment and differential diagnosis of schizophrenia and bipolar disorder can be challenging for family physicians and other healthcare professionals. Since psychotic symptoms occur in both schizophrenia and bipolar disorder, it can be easy to confuse the two diagnoses. In addition, schizophrenia and bipolar disorder can be difficult to distinguish from one another when patients, family members and other healthcare professionals give vague descriptions of symptoms, such as 'behaves oddly' or 'has mood swings.' Establishing the history and diagnosis can be further complicated in the absence of medical/psychiatric records to serve as supportive documentation. Finally, healthcare providers need to rule out organic etiology, substance abuse and other psychiatric disorders in order to make the correct diagnosis.

Primary care providers can provide the initial diagnosis and treatment of schizophrenia/bipolar disorder, as well as continuity of care for patients with established diagnoses. The movie clips described in this chapter can help learners to become more familiar with the presentation and treatment of individuals who suffer with these conditions.

## Schizophrenia

### Public perceptions of people with schizophrenia

◆ *The Caveman's Valentine* (Samuel L Jackson, Ann Magnuson, Aunjanue Ellis). This is the story of Romulus Ledbetter (Samuel L Jackson), an accomplished pianist, who experiences persecutory and paranoid delusions as well as auditory and visual hallucinations. Romulus is homeless, lives in a rocky enclosure/cave in a New York City park and is known to locals as 'the Caveman.' Romulus becomes preoccupied with the death of a young homeless man he once knew, and seeks to learn the truth behind his death. Due to his history of mental health problems, those around him simply believe he is acting 'crazy' once again.

a (0:01:42–0:02:48). In this opening scene Romulus is in the midst of a public tirade on the street. There is a police officer close by, ready for action if things get out of hand. Romulus says loudly to those around him 'Don't you watch me.'

b (0:04:04–0:06:40). Romulus asks a passer-by if he can borrow a pencil. The passer-by strikes up a conversation with Romulus and is surprised to see him writing music. When Romulus tells him that he went to the Juilliard School of Music, the man asks how he ended up on the street. This triggers an outburst from Romulus involving his primary persecutory figure, Stiverson, a fictitious man who lives at the top of the Chrysler building. Romulus believes that Stiverson watches him and is trying to take over the world. Romulus's rambling triggers an auditory hallucination.

1 What do these scenes communicate about people who are homeless?
2 What do these scenes communicate about homeless people who have a mental illness?
3 How would you handle a patient who becomes loud and angry during an outpatient visit?
4 What are some guidelines with regard to handling possible endangerment in the office?
5 What is the best way to approach someone like Romulus who is agitated?

## Symptoms of schizophrenia

### Lack of social connection with or interest in others

◆ *A Beautiful Mind* (Russell Crowe, Jennifer Connelly, Ed Harris). This movie is based on the life of the Nobel Prize-winning mathematician John Nash (Russell Crowe). He is considered odd and socially awkward in graduate school, yet his schizophrenia remains hidden until the day he runs out of his own lecture and is involuntarily hospitalized. The film chronicles the impact of the illness on John and his wife, Alicia (Jennifer Connelly), his many attempts to solve his schizophrenia on his own and his efforts to stay connected to his life despite his illness. Two of the most interesting aspects of this film are its depiction of how schizophrenia can remain undetected for years and its portrayal of the schizophrenic's internal experience.

a (0:33:38–0:34:04). John is getting oriented to his new job. We find out later in the film that the figure (Ed Harris) to whom he is talking is a delusion. It is noted that John has neither family nor friends. John senses that other people do not like him, but he minimizes their feelings: 'I like to think it's because I'm a lone wolf.'

1 How would you respond to a parent who was concerned that their child was 'a loner'?
2 What questions would you ask to assess severe social isolation?
3 How would you respond if, during a brief assessment of social support, a patient stated 'I don't have any close friends'?

### Visual hallucinations

◆ *A Beautiful Mind* (Russell Crowe, Jennifer Connelly, Ed Harris). See previous section on lack of social connection with or interest in others for movie description.

a (1:07:00–1:09:20). John is in a psychiatric hospital talking with his psychiatrist. The psychiatrist realizes that John is responding to some visual stimuli and says, 'Tell me who you see.' John thinks that he sees his graduate-school roommate, Charles, and engages in a dialogue with him.

b (1:36:15–1:38:16). This clip includes more examples of auditory, visual and command hallucinations occurring before, during and after John is supposed to be giving his baby a bath. He is confused and threatening to other people.

1 What are some indications (e.g. behavioral observations) that a patient is responding to fictitious internal/visual stimuli?
2 Which type of hallucination – auditory or visual – is most characteristic of schizophrenia? (Auditory hallucinations are by far the most common type and most characteristic of schizophrenia. The film depicts many non-reality-based visual images, which may be used to assist the audience in experiencing John Nash's internal state of being.)

## Paranoia/paranoid behavior

◆ *A Beautiful Mind* (Russell Crowe, Jennifer Connelly, Ed Harris). See earlier section on lack of social connection with or interest in others for movie description.

a (1:14:36–1:17:15). Alicia visits John in the psychiatric hospital. Initially he appears quite 'normal' as he reassures his wife that everything will be fine. However, soon he exhibits paranoid behavior and says 'They may be listening' and 'There may be microphones.' His wife tells him 'It isn't real. There's no conspiracy. It's in your mind.'

1 How would you respond to a patient who displayed paranoid delusions like John's?
2 Would you take the approach depicted by John's wife? Why or why not?
3 How do you feel when you are in the presence of patients with paranoid delusions? What reactions do they elicit from you? What reactions do they elicit from others?

## Pressured, unintelligible speech

◆ *Shine* (Geoffrey Rush, Lynn Redgrave, John Gielgud). This is the true story of David Helfgott (Geoffrey Rush), a gifted pianist, who grows up being physically and emotionally abused by his intrusive and controlling father. While David's exact diagnosis is deliberately left vague, it is clear that he was damaged by his upbringing. Following a mental breakdown, David does not resume his previous level of functioning.

a (0:0:03–0:05:15). In this scene, David walks into a restaurant and speaks at a rapid, unintelligible pace while people around him look on in amazement.

1 How would you characterize David's speech?
2 How would you respond to a patient who, like David, presents with rapid, unintelligible speech in the office?
3 What would you say to family members or staff members who ask why a patient, like David, is speaking in a rapid, unintelligible way?

## Self-destructive behavior in response to a delusional belief

◆ *A Beautiful Mind* (Russell Crowe, Jennifer Connelly, Ed Harris). See earlier section on lack of social connection with or interest in others for movie description.

**a** (1:17:14–1:20:26). John is being viewed from the observation room. He has cut his arm and is bleeding. Code red is called at the psychiatric hospital. John's behavior stems from his desire to rid himself of an implant that he believes is in his arm. He states in disbelief that 'The implant is gone. I can't find it.' He receives electroconvulsive therapy (ECT).

1   How do you access emergency mental healthcare in the outpatient setting?
2   What safeguards should be instituted to protect mentally ill patients and others?
3   What is your reaction to electroconvulsive therapy? When is such therapy warranted?

## Patient description of the experience/symptoms

◆ *The Caveman's Valentine* (Samuel L Jackson, Ann Magnuson, Aunjanue Ellis). See earlier section on public perceptions of people with schizophrenia for movie description.

**a** (0:52:50–0:53:58). Romulus is outside a guesthouse, looking in. Inside the dog barks and we see a woman that he has just met. She looks towards the window to see Romulus peering through and following a moment of apprehension, invites him in. Based on his behavior at a dinner party they attended earlier that evening, she asks him if he is psychotic. Romulus responds 'I have brain typhoons, swarms of moths howling in my skull.'

1   How would you explain schizophrenia to a patient?

## Treating the family of a schizophrenic patient

### Educating the family about the diagnosis and reactions to the diagnosis

◆ *A Beautiful Mind* (Russell Crowe, Jennifer Connelly, Ed Harris). See earlier section on lack of social connection with or interest in others for movie description.

**a** (1:09:22–1:11:39). In this scene the psychiatrist breaks the news to Mrs Nash (Jennifer Connelly) that her husband has schizophrenia. She initially displays disbelief, until she is confronted with the overwhelming evidence of her husband's significant mental deterioration.

**b** (1:11:42–1:13:06). Alicia Nash goes to her husband's office to gather information about his work and look for clues about his illness. She sees at first hand that her husband's 'work' revolves around cutting out magazine pictures with government/spy themes and posting them on the walls of his office. Colleagues admit to not knowing about John's work, and comment that 'lately he'd become more agitated.'

1   What questions and issues are family members likely to have about a loved one who is diagnosed with schizophrenia or another serious psychiatric disorder?
2   What can you do to educate families about mental illness?
3   What would you say to a family member who asked you about the root cause of schizophrenia?
4   How would you respond to a 30-year-old woman whose mother has schizo-

phrenia, and wonders if she could develop the disorder? How would you respond if the daughter was 19 years old?

## Family coping over time

- *A Beautiful Mind* (Russell Crowe, Jennifer Connelly, Ed Harris). See earlier section on lack of social connection with or interest in others for movie description.

a (1:20:50–1:22:22). About a year after John's diagnosis, a friend asks his wife how she is holding up. She describes an array of emotions, including obligation, guilt about wanting to leave the marriage, and rage.

1 If Alicia Nash was your patient, what advice or guidance about coping could you give her?
2 How do you feel about Mrs Nash's emotional reaction to her husband's disorder?
3 What resources could you make available to Mrs Nash to help her to cope with her husband's schizophrenia?

## Non-adherence

- *A Beautiful Mind* (Russell Crowe, Jennifer Connelly, Ed Harris). See earlier section on lack of connection with or interest in others for movie description.

a (1:39:00–1:41:10). In this scene John explains to his psychiatrist why he has stopped taking his medications. He says 'All I have to do is control my thinking.'

1 Discuss different approaches to handling medication non-adherence in patients. How might your approach differ in managing non-adherence in patients with psychiatric illness?
2 What are some potential benefits of primary care collaboration with a patient's psychiatrist?

# Bipolar disorder

## Mania

- *Mr Jones* (Richard Gere, Lena Olin, Anne Bancroft). This is the story of a 35-year-old man, Mr Jones (Richard Gere), with bipolar disorder. The film demonstrates his manic episodes, depressive spirals and crashes, interactions with the psychiatric community and difficulty adhering to a medication regimen.

a (0:06:50–0:10:02). Mr Jones has just walked onto a construction project. He is in an expansive, elevated mood. He gives 100 dollars to someone he has just met and then climbs onto a thin steel beam, asking 'Do you feel like flying?'. A co-worker is concerned for Mr Jones and warns him not to go any further. Mr Jones rambles on about physics and equilibrium as an ambulance approaches to take him away.

b (0:19:33–0:24:10). Mr Jones closes a bank account that he opened five days earlier. He gives 100 dollars to the teller and asks her out to lunch. They go to a piano store and he buys a piano. Then they go to a hotel room. After disrupting a symphony performance, Mr Jones is apprehended by the police.

1 Why is mania such a dangerous condition?
2 What are some different ways in which hypomanic/manic patients present to healthcare professionals?
3 What are effective treatments for mania?

## Assessment/mental status

### Psychiatry rounds/misdiagnosis

◆ *Mr Jones* (Richard Gere, Lena Olin, Anna Bancroft). See previous section on mania for movie description.

a (0:10:16–0:12:50). The psychiatrists and residents conduct rounds. Some residents are being oriented to the hospital's 'cut-off policy (evaluate–medicate–vacate).' The chief psychiatrist (Lena Olin) highlights the importance of evaluating the patient's orientation immediately upon arrival. Someone describes how Mr Jones arrived at the hospital highly agitated, delusional and having auditory hallucinations. A preliminary working diagnosis of paranoid schizophrenia is given.

1 What do you think about the hospital's 'cut-off policy'?
2 What do you know about the constraints on the psychiatric inpatient services available in your community?

## Clarification of the diagnosis

◆ *Mr Jones* (Richard Gere, Lena Olin, Anne Bancroft). See earlier section on mania for movie description.

a (0:16:08–0:19:15). As he leaves the hospital, Mr Jones sexualizes his interaction with his psychiatrist. She has not had an opportunity to interview him formally, and at a staff meeting she states that Mr Jones was misdiagnosed and is manic. She adds that he is psychotic and not schizophrenic, describing him as 'expansive, intrusive and euphoric.'

1 What does this clip reveal about the assessment process? What does it reveal about the need sometimes for multiple clinical observations?

### Discussing the diagnosis with a patient

◆ *Mr Jones* (Richard Gere, Lena Olin, Anne Bancroft). See earlier section on mania for movie description.

a (0:27:20–0:30:52). Mr Jones is brought to the hospital after a frenetic day. He is agitated as his doctor explains to him that he has manic-depressive disorder. The doctor says it is like having diabetes, and Mr Jones tells him it is not an illness but 'who I am.' He says 'I like who I am.'

1 How would you respond to this statement by Mr Jones?
2 How would you explain the diagnosis of bipolar disorder to a patient and to a member of their family?

3   What is the difference between mania and hypomania? What questions would you ask to distinguish between the two disorders?

4   What symptom is most diagnostic of mania?

5   What is it about their condition that bipolar patients like?

## Descent into depression

◆ *Mr Jones* (Richard Gere, Lena Olin, Anne Bancroft). See earlier section on mania for movie description.

a   (0:45:36–0:47:52). Mr Jones is at the construction site from which he had previously been taken away by ambulance. A man he had met there talks to him and invites him over for dinner to pick up his tools. At dinner, his friend notices that Mr Jones is not his previous 'upbeat' self. As Mr Jones walks into the bedroom of his friend's child, we see how physically slowed down he has become as he struggles to help the child with a maths problem.

b   (0:47:56–0:49:45). Mr Jones has auditory hallucinations as he walks through a music school and looks into the various rooms. He walks dangerously close to cars and we see his disheveled appearance.

c   (0:49:46–0:52:03). The friend from the construction site tracks down Mr Jones' psychiatrist and explains that he is concerned about Mr Jones. The psychiatrist then tries to locate him. When they eventually meet up, Mr Jones is walking the streets. He cries in front of his psychiatrist and says 'I can't stop the sadness.'

d   (0:52:04–0:52:26). After Mr Jones is admitted to hospital he is showered and sung to by a psychiatric aide. He appears physically and mentally depleted.

e   (0:52:27–0:53:34). Mr Jones is talking with his psychiatrist and explains that he and his father had a fight. The psychiatrist tells him that they are dealing with two problems – the chemical one for which Mr Jones is being treated, and another one related to his emotional pain. The psychiatrist attempts to get a commitment from Mr Jones to work together.

1   What are the risks of a patient remaining untreated during a depressive phase?

2   How would you advise a family member who calls you, concerned about a loved one being so despondent?

## Reaction to the medication regimen

◆ *Mr Jones* (Richard Gere, Lena Olin, Anne Bancroft). See earlier section on mania for movie description.

a   (1:08:50–1:12:20). Mr Jones talks with his psychiatrist about missing his high moods. He states 'I am a junkie. I need me. I really miss my highs.' He sadly admits 'I'm not normal.'

1   How would you respond to Mr Jones' statements?

# Chapter 15

# Personality and dissociative disorders

*Jay C Williams and Matthew Alexander*

In Chapter 19, four types of 'hateful' patients are described, namely 'dependent clingers', 'entitled demanders', 'manipulative help rejecters' and 'self-destructive deniers'.[1] In this chapter, the authors add five types of difficult patients to Groves' typology. These represent common features of certain personality disorders and dissociative disorders. They are emotionally over-reactive patients, self-centered patients, dishonest patients, eccentric patients and patients who dissociate. This behaviorally focused typology may be easier for learners to grasp than more technical labels.

## Personality disorders

What is a personality disorder? Personality disorders are enduring, stable and culturally dystonic patterns of thought, feeling and action that cause distress and/ or impaired functioning.[2] Personality disorders have overlapping characteristics and may manifest as mixed types or be comorbid with other mental conditions such as mood disorders, anxiety disorders or substance-related disorders. Although personality disorders can be difficult to differentiate, they are divided into 'clusters' that are more distinct. Cluster A consists of the odd, eccentric type (paranoid, schizoid and schizotypal). Cluster B consists of the dramatic, emotional, erratic type (antisocial, borderline, histrionic and narcissistic). Cluster C consists of the anxious, fearful type (avoidant, dependent and obsessive-compulsive). A fourth category, personality disorders not otherwise specified (NOS), includes all personality disorders not included in the other clusters (passive–aggressive, sadomasochistic, etc.). Not all patients with personality disorders are 'hateful' in Groves' terms, but the cluster B personality disorders, together with paranoid and dependent personality disorders, correspond to Groves' types.

While individuals with personality disorders may constitute a minority of patients seen in most healthcare practices, they can consume inordinate amounts of a clinician's energy if not properly identified and treated. Since the diagnosis of personality disorders is something that occurs over time and is easy to miss in practice, movie clips are a particularly useful way to help learners to 'see' what people with personality disorders 'look like' so that they can make earlier and more accurate diagnoses.

### Emotionally over-reactive patients

Emotionally over-reactive patients can turn what would normally be a reasonable doctor–patient interaction into an uproar. Rage, panic and high drama are characteristic of all cluster B personality disorders. An excellent cinematic example of this type of individual is found in the Glenn Close character in *Fatal Attraction* (see section on dependent clingers' in Chapter 19).

◆ *Girl, Interrupted* (Winona Ryder, Angelina Jolie, Whoopie Goldberg, Vanessa Redgrave). This is a film adaptation of Susanna Kaysen's autobiographical book about her hospitalization for borderline personality disorder.

a (1:10:50–1:19:02). This scene shows Susanna (Winona Ryder) talking with Dr Wick (Vanessa Redgrave) about her condition, panicking when her friend is missing, and becoming enraged at Nurse Valerie (Whoopie Goldberg).

1 What features of borderline personality disorder does Susanna demonstrate?
2 Have you known a patient, friend or relative who has shown similar traits?
3 How might such emotional reactivity be managed?

◆ *A Streetcar Named Desire* (Vivien Leigh, Marlon Brando). This film, based on the play by Tennessee Williams, depicts the interaction between histrionic Blanche (Vivien Leigh), who tenaciously holds on to the belief that she will soon be returned to the finer life she deserves, and her brutish brother-in-law, Stanley (Marlon Brando).

a (1:39:30–1:41:21). This scene shows Stanley and Blanche talking about an 'old beau' while Stanley awaits the birth of his child.

1 What characteristics of histrionic personality disorder does Blanche illustrate?
2 What feelings does she evoke in you?
3 Can you think of patients or individuals in your personal life who were similarly histrionic?
4 What are some ways to manage histrionic behaviors in your patients?

## Self-centered patients

It is difficult to like patients who are extremely self-centered, who feel entitled to special treatment and who become enraged when they do not get what they want. Rage or instantaneous and disproportionate anger is common among all cluster B personality disorders. Another trait common to these individuals is an absence of empathy for others' suffering.

◆ *What About Bob?* (Bill Murray, Richard Dreyfuss). This dark but very funny movie tells the story of Bob Wiley (Bill Murray), a highly anxious individual who invades the personal life of his therapist, Dr Leo Marvin (Richard Dreyfuss).

a (0:07:11–0:11:40). Bob uses flattery to manipulate and 'hook' Dr Marvin into taking him on as a patient. Dr Marvin's narcissism makes him very susceptible.

1 What elements of narcissistic personality disorder are revealed by Dr Marvin in this clip?
2 What useful distinctions can be made between having a full-blown personality disorder and personality traits?
3 Have you encountered narcissistic individuals in either your professional or personal life? How do you feel in the presence of such individuals? Can you distinguish between 'healthy' and 'pathological' narcissism?

4 How is Bob able to 'hook' Dr Marvin into taking him on as a patient? How are overblown statements about a provider, often made during an initial contact, a 'tip-off' of possible cluster B personality disorder? What is the best way for a provider to handle such unrealistic praise?

◆ *Citizen Kane* (Orson Welles, Joseph Cotton, Agnes Moorehead). This classic film chronicles the drive of Charles Foster Kane (Orson Welles) for power, wealth and fame, and his inability to care about others.

a (1:42:46–1:45:51). When Kane's wife leaves him, he responds with narcissistic rage and physical abuse. He is unable to care about her, and only concerns himself with what other people will think.

1 What aspects of narcissistic personality disorder does Kane manifest?
2 Why does he become so enraged?
3 What feelings does Kane evoke in you?
4 Have you known a patient, friend, relative or acquaintance who was similarly narcissistic?
5 What are some ways to handle narcissistic behavior in your patients?

## Dishonest patients

How can you take a reliable history from a patient who lies? It is characteristic of patients with antisocial personality disorder to trust no one and to say whatever they believe will get them what they want. Similarly, patients with addictions may lie and manipulate in order to support their addiction. It is often hard to tell whether their behavior is the result of a personality disorder or a substance-related disorder. Over time, the behaviors of an addict may become so much a part of their personality that their origin becomes moot.

◆ *Dead Man Walking* (Susan Sarandon, Sean Penn). This film is based on Sister Helen Prejean's autobiographical book about her experience serving as a spiritual counselor to convicted murderer, Matthew Poncelet.

a (0:08:05–0:13:11). Sister Helen (Susan Sarandon) meets Matthew (Sean Penn), and it becomes clear that he lies, feels no remorse and trusts no one.

1 Why has Matthew become mistrustful, dishonest, remorseless and violent?
2 Is there any goodness left in Matthew? If so, can you think of ways to find it and bring it out in him?
3 Do you know a patient, friend, relative or acquaintance who shows similar, if less extreme, antisocial traits? If so, how do you feel in their presence?
4 How could you ensure your own safety and work effectively with a patient like Matthew?

◆ *Jungle Fever* (Wesley Snipes, Annabella Sciorra, Samuel L Jackson, Ruby Dee, Ossie Davis). This is one of Spike Lee's films about race relations.

a (0:21:40–0:24:12). Gator (Samuel L Jackson), a heroin addict, lies and charms his mother into giving him money to support his addiction.

1 What causes Gator's ruthlessness?

2 How can you think about Gator's addiction in such a way as to regard him positively?
3 Have you ever known patients, friends or relatives with a substance abuse problem?
4 What are some things you can do to work effectively with a patient who has a substance abuse problem?

## Eccentric patients

Occasionally patients are cooperative, but so shy or eccentric that it is hard to establish a relationship with them. Such patients can be introverted and avoid seeking the medical care that they need, or may be reticent in describing their concerns. They may also present bizarre and perplexing concerns. The personality disorders that are characterized by such odd behavior include avoidant, paranoid, schizoid and schizotypal disorders.

◆ *Annie Hall* (Woody Allen, Diane Keaton). This Academy Award-winning movie tells the story of Alvy Singer (Woody Allen), a New York comic, and his girlfriend, Annie (Diane Keaton).

a (0:47:15–0:48:45). In this hilarious but disturbing scene, Annie's brother Dwayne (Christopher Walken) tells Alvy about a bizarre obsession. The scene follows a family Thanksgiving meal in which Annie's extended family meets Alvy for the first time.

1 What characteristics of schizotypal personality disorder are displayed by Dwayne? How would you distinguish between schizotypal personality disorder and schizoid personality disorder?
2 Have you ever worked with or known individuals similar to Dwayne?
3 What types of feeling do individuals with schizotypal or schizoid personality disorder typically evoke in their caregivers?
4 What is the best way to provide care for someone with a schizotypal or schizoid personality disorder?

◆ *Unstrung Heroes* (Nathan Watt, Andie McDowell, John Turturro, Michael Richards, Maury Chaykin). This touching and funny film concerns the struggles of two eccentric uncles caring for their nephew Stephen (Nathan Watt), who moves in with them when his mother (Andie McDowell) develops cancer. The paranoia displayed by Danny (Michael Richards) is characteristic of a paranoid personality disorder or delusional disorder. The literal thinking and eccentricity displayed by Arthur (Maury Chaykin) are characteristic of schizotypal personality disorder.

a (0:14:41–0:18:24). This scene depicts a family gathering in which Danny's paranoia upsets everyone and Arthur tenderly offers his sister-in-law a 'remedy' made from junk he has collected.

1 What oddities of thought and behavior do Arthur and Danny display?
2 What impact do the two uncles have on the extended family? Can you generalize to all families with mentally ill relatives?
3 What kinds of clinical problem might patients like Arthur and Danny present to their physician?

4  How might Arthur's problems be managed?

5  How might Danny's problems be managed?

## Dissociative disorders

Dissociative disorders are those in which part of one's identity is experienced as split off, unreal or unremembered.[2] Popular usage misleadingly refers to schizophrenia as a *split personality*. In fact, schizophrenia is a disorder in which various mental functions and aspects of personality *deteriorate*, and it is not to be confused with dissociative disorders. The most extreme dissociative disorder is dissociative identity disorder, formerly known as multiple personality disorder. However, there are other less dramatic forms of dissociation, such as fugue states, amnesia and feelings of unreality.

The problem with treating a patient with a dissociative disorder is knowing with whom one is speaking. Dissociative disorders involve discontinuity of experience, such that a patient may not remember or 'own' what they have done on another occasion. For obvious reasons, this complicates both accurate reporting of medical history and reliable follow-through of medical recommendations.

◆  *Never Talk to Strangers* (Rebecca DeMornay, Antonio Banderas). This is a suspenseful film about a previously abused woman, Dr Sarah Taylor (Rebecca DeMornay), who develops dissociative identity disorder.

a  (1:09:22–1:19:47). In this climactic scene, Sarah's various alter egos (i.e. personalities) are revealed.

1  Have you ever been acquainted with a patient, friend or relative who experienced significant or less dramatic forms of dissociation?

2  What is the role of Sarah's prior emotional and sexual abuse in the development of her dissociative identity disorder?

3  How might you obtain accurate medical information and ensure reliable follow-up of dissociative patients?

## Conclusion

Personality disorders and dissociative disorders complicate the diagnosis and treatment of patients. However, such patients can be rewarding to work with if one understands their personality aberrations as maladaptive attempts to cope with difficult life events, and if one can be creative in finding ways to accommodate these aberrations.

## References

1.  Groves J. Taking care of the hateful patient. *NEJM* 1978; **298**: 883–7.
2.  APA. *DSM-IV-TR: diagnostic and statistical manual of mental disorders* (4e). Washington, DC: American Psychiatric Association, 2001.

# Chapter 16

# Eating disorders

*Patricia Lenahan, Anna Pavlov and Matthew Alexander*

Family physicians are likely to encounter patients with the full gamut of eating disorders in their practices, ranging from patients with body image disturbances to those who need to maintain an unhealthy weight in order to participate in dance or athletics, and those who engage in emotional and compulsive eating. Identification and treatment of eating disorders may be a complicated process that involves not only the individual but also the family. Treatment is complicated due to the special psychological, ethnic and cultural meanings of food. Ideally, physicians should be aware of such complicating factors when counseling individuals about eating disorders. The video clips discussed in this chapter focus primarily on obesity, a serious condition that predisposes individuals to developing heart disease, hypertension, hypercholesterolemia and diabetes.

## Obesity

### Childhood obesity

◆ *Lovely and Amazing* (Catherine Keener, Emily Mortimer, Brenda Blethyn, Raven Goodwin). This film depicts a family of women who are navigating jobs and personal roles, and who struggle with societal expectations regarding physical traits. The Caucasian matriarch, Jane Marks (Brenda Blethyn), has two grown-up daughters and an adopted 8-year-old African-American girl, Annie (Raven Goodwin), who is overweight and 'inherits' some of her family's insecurities and values. The matriarch undergoes plastic surgery with complications.

a (1:18:56–1:22:40). Annie's adult sister walks into a McDonald's fast-food restaurant and is surprised to see Annie there alone with a trayful of food. She realizes that they have all inherited their mother's insecurities despite being 'lovely and amazing.'

1 How consistently do you counsel parents of overweight children or talk with teenagers about weight management?
2 Why do you think such counseling does not occur more frequently in practice?
3 What barriers exist to counseling parents/teenagers about weight management?
4 How can you and your staff work with/around such barriers?
5 What would make weight management of children and adolescents an easier topic to discuss?

6 What cultural and ethnic factors should you consider when addressing issues related to food?
7 What is the relationship between fast-food consumption, economic stress and obesity?
8 How would you counsel a family with regard to the amount of fast food in their diet?

## Social judgements about obesity

◆ *What's Eating Gilbert Grape?* (Johnny Depp, Leonardo DiCaprio, Mary Steenburgen, Juliette Lewis). This movie tells the story of the Grape family, who live in the small rural community of Endora. This single-parent household consists of a morbidly obese mother (Darlene Cates), her mentally impaired son Arnie (Leonardo DiCaprio), his caretaking brother Gilbert (Johnny Depp) and their two sisters, Amy and Ellen. Juliette Lewis plays the out-of-town visitor who changes Gilbert's life.

a (01:05:02–01:07:52). In this scene, Bonnie Grape (Darlene Cates), the morbidly obese matriarch of the Grape family, who has not ventured outside the family home in seven years, is taken by her children to the police station to retrieve her son Arnie (Leonardo DiCaprio) out of jail. Her excessive weight prompts considerable gawking by a crowd of bystanders.

1 Do you think that this scene exaggerates the degree of negative reactions encountered by morbidly obese individuals?
2 How do you understand people's negative reactions to overweight individuals?
3 What are your negative reactions, if any, to overweight patients?
4 What type of concurrent psychiatric diagnoses may be present in individuals with disordered eating?
5 What are effective treatment strategies to help motivated patients to lose weight?

## Familial influences on obesity

◆ *Heavy* (Shelley Winters, Deborah Harry, Liv Tyler, Pruitt Taylor Vincent). Victor (Pruitt Taylor Vincent) is an overweight cook who lives with his domineering mother, Dolly (Shelley Winters), and works in her diner. Victor becomes attracted to the new waitress, Callie (Liv Tyler), whom his mother has just hired. Victor, a virgin, begins to fantasize about Callie, which frightens Dolly, who fears that she is losing control over her son.

a (0:30:00–0:31:15). The scene begins with Victor weighing himself and the scale registering 250 pounds. It then shifts to Dolly sitting at the breakfast table and complaining that everything hurts. She chides Victor for skipping his breakfast – 'the most important meal of the day'. Victor replies that he is fat. Dolly tells him that he is 'husky, well-built and macho.'

1 What is the impact of the family on eating patterns and behaviors?
2 What factors, other than hunger, might be motivating Victor's desire to eat?

3   What is the impact of Dolly's denial of Victor's statement that he is fat?
4   What is the purpose of her calling him husky and well-built as opposed to fat?

## Compulsive overeating

◆ *Fatso* (Dom Deluise, Anne Bancroft, Candice Azzara). This movie, directed by Anne Bancroft, tells the story of Dominick DiNapoli (Dom Deluise), an overweight man who is nagged by his sister (Anne Bancroft) to lose weight after the sudden death of an obese cousin. The movie is alternately very funny and touching.

a   (0:00:00–0:06:36). The sequence of scenes begins with a series of snapshots of DiNapoli's food-oriented childhood, and then moves to the DiNapoli family grieving the sudden death of an obese cousin.

1   How can early experiences with food impact on childhood and adult obesity?
2   What are cultural patterns related to eating?
3   What are the various meanings that food has for people (e.g. love, comfort, etc.)?
4   How can you successfully treat someone who eats for emotional reasons?

b   (1:23:38–1:27:20). Feeling rejected by his girlfriend, Lydia (Candice Azzara), DiNapoli goes on a binge, disappearing from his family to gorge on Chinese take-out food. In this clip, DiNapoli is confronted by his sister and comes to terms with his life-long legacy of eating. He pleads for his brother and sister to accept him for 'who I am.'

1   What does this scene illustrate about emotional eating? What does it illustrate about the influence of family-of-origin issues on obesity?
2   If DiNapoli was your patient, how would you counsel him about dealing with this relapse?
3   What does this scene reveal about the need for individuals to maintain self-consistency (the motivation to be the same person today that one was yesterday)?
4   As a healthcare professional, how would you respond to an obese patient who wants to be accepted 'as they are'?

## Anorexia/bulimia

◆ *Center Stage* (Peter Gallagher, Susan May Pratt). This is a film about the competitive life of professional dancers in New York City.

a   (1:13:30–1:17:20). When her boyfriend confronts Maureen about throwing up everything she eats, she explodes and denies that she has a problem.

1   In what ways do anorexia and bulimia present to medical professionals?
2   What is the best way to screen for these disorders?
3   How do you understand the level of denial shown by Maureen in this clip?
4   What type of interdisciplinary approach works best when treating eating-disordered patients?
5   Have you ever had, or known anyone else who has had, an eating disorder?

# Body image

◆ *Real Women Have Curves* (America Ferrera, Lupe Ontiveros, Ingrid Olin, George Lopez, Brian Sites). Ana (America Ferrera) is an overweight teenager who has just graduated from Beverly Hills High School. With the encouragement of one of her teachers (George Lopez), Ana pursues her dreams of attending college and receives a full scholarship to Columbia. However, her mother has other ideas. She wants Ana to work in the dress factory of her older sister Estela (Ingrid Olin).

a (1:09:21–1:13:49). Ana is working in her sister's factory. She is ironing, feeling hot and takes off her shirt. Her mother tells her that she looks awful and should put her shirt back on. Ana tells her mother that she likes herself, and her sister Estela agrees. Her mother tells her that they are both fat. Ana tells her mother that she is fat, too. Her mother says that that is okay because she is married. This leads to a discussion of appearances, weight and cellulite. All of the women begin taking off their clothes and comparing sizes, stretch marks and cellulite. They all say they are beautiful. Ana adds 'this is who we are.' The scene ends with all the women continuing to work and dance in their underwear.

1   What impact do parents' judgements have on a child's body image?
2   What is the relationship between body image and self-esteem for women and also increasingly for men?

# Cosmetic surgery (liposuction)

◆ *Lovely and Amazing* (Catherine Keener, Emily Mortimer, Brenda Blethyn, Raven Goodwin). See earlier section on childhood obesity for movie description.

a (0:28:56–0:30:56). There are postoperative complications as Jane (Brenda Blethyn) feels nauseous and in pain. She voices regret about undergoing the surgery because she hurts so much. The surgeon reassures her that she will feel better soon. She will need to stay in hospital overnight because of dehydration. Her physician tells her that he removed 'ten pounds of fat' and he thinks she will be very pleased with the results.

1   What are the postoperative complications of liposuction?
2   What are your personal feelings about liposuction?
3   How would you counsel a patient who is interested in undergoing liposuction?

# Part IV

## The doctor–patient relationship

# Chapter 17

# Interviewing skills

*Dael Waxman, Matthew Alexander, Heather A Kirkpatrick*
*and Pablo Gonzalez Blasco*

Intuitively, it is well understood that good communicators make good healthcare professionals. In fact, physicians with excellent communication skills have long been said to possess 'a good bedside manner.' This intuitive awareness that communication is important in medicine has been supported by research results. Empirically, effective communication skills of clinicians have been shown[1-4] to lead to improved:

1 accuracy in the identification of patient problems
2 patient satisfaction
3 patient adherence to treatment recommendations (and therefore improved clinical outcomes)
4 patient understanding of clinical problems and treatment options.

Historically, attention to clinical interviewing in medical education has often been absent or haphazard. However, given the empirical findings, attention is now increasingly being given to communication skills training in healthcare. Several models of effective communication curricula have been proposed, tested and taught. In recent years, proponents of various strategies have achieved consensus about which specific interviewing skills have a positive influence on clinical outcomes.[5] The selected clips in this chapter highlight some of those skills as well as some non-exemplary approaches to interviewing. It is our experience that viewing the communication techniques demonstrated by these clips greatly enhances the interviewing skills curriculum.

## Active listening

◆ *Patch Adams* (Robin Williams). This is a movie based on the true story of Dr Hunter 'Patch' Adams (Robin Williams) and his experiences during medical school. Despite the emphasis on objectivity in medical culture, Patch tries to bring warmth and healing to his interactions with patients, challenging the status quo by interacting with patients in unconventional ways.

a (0:05:18–0:06:50). In this scene, Patch is being interviewed by a psychiatrist concurrent with his voluntary admission to a psychiatric institution. Patch bares his soul but the psychiatrist appears to be uninterested, neither making eye contact nor appearing to really listen to what Patch is saying.

1 What specific examples of ineffective active listening occur in this clip?

2  If you were giving feedback to the physician about his interviewing skills, what would you tell him?
3  How would you imagine Patch feels during this encounter?
4  Have you seen this type of ineffective listening in the practice of medicine?
5  What types of patient or problem cause *you* to 'tune out' as a physician?

## Rapport building

◆ *Patch Adams* (Robin Williams). See previous section on active listening for movie description.

a (0:25:03–0:26:10). Here we see Patch making a connection with an inpatient with diabetes after an impersonal, 'objective' and insensitive presentation of the patient by an attending physician.

1  How might the attending physician's case presentation have been conducted more compassionately?
2  Why is rapport building important in the physician–patient encounter?
3  How have you dealt with situations in which you witnessed a non-humanistic approach in medicine but felt disempowered to address it?

b (0:43:30–0:44:54, 0:50:13–0:52:05). In these two scenes, Patch visits a patient who is notorious for being 'difficult.' By taking an unconventional approach, Patch achieves meaningful patient rapport.

1  What is Patch's first reaction to the patient's aggressiveness? What would your first reaction be?
2  What patient emotion does Patch seem to 'hear' on an unspoken level?
3  How does listening on an emotional level alter our relationships with patients and impact our interviewing?

## Non-verbal communication

◆ *Awakenings* (Robin Williams). This movie tells the true story of Dr Oliver Sacks, who in the film is named Dr Malcolm Sayer (Robin Williams). After years of research work, Dr Sayer takes his first clinical neurology position. Once he is in his new position, Dr Sayer begins innovative treatment of post-encephalitis patients using L-dopa, causing patients to 'awaken' from long-term comas.

a (0:11:15–0:12:20). In this clip, Dr Sayer conducts an initial interview with Lucy, a non-responsive patient.

1  How might *you* have coped in this interview with Lucy?
2  Despite the fact that he suspects Lucy cannot comprehend him, Dr Sayer still shows concern for her. How does he communicate this concern?
3  Discuss the importance of non-verbal communication in human interaction.
4  How aware are you of your own non-verbal communication with patients?
5  How do cultural differences impact non-verbal communication with patients?

# The patient-centered approach

◆ *The Doctor* (William Hurt, Wendy Crewson, Christine Lahti). This is a powerful movie about an insensitive surgeon who battles throat cancer and has a 'change of heart' that makes him act more compassionately towards patients and his family.

a (0:09:30–0:10:26). Dr McGee (William Hurt) conducts a 'chart-focused' interview with a woman who has undergone chest surgery.

1 How would this interview be different if it were 'patient centered' rather than 'chart centered'?
2 What are the advantages and disadvantages of the 'physician-centered' interview?
3 What are the advantages and disadvantages of the 'patient-centered' interview?

b (0:20:03–0:23:47). Dr McGee goes to see Dr Leslie Abbott (Wendy Crewson), a throat surgeon, for an evaluation. Dr Abbott diagnoses Dr McGee as having a malignant tumour.

1 What aspects of this interview are dealt with well? What aspects of the interview could be improved?
2 How could you use this clip to distinguish between a physician-centered and a patient-centered approach to the medical interview?

◆ *The Legend of 1900* (Tim Roth). This brilliant movie tells the story of the world's most gifted pianist, named '1900,' who has never left the ocean liner on which he was born in the year 1900.

a (0:50:00–0:52:40). In this scene, 1900 explains to another musician that much of his musical inspiration comes from closely observing people.

1 What can you learn from this scene about becoming more patient centered in your work?
2 How can you avoid letting scheduling issues and too narrow a focus on diagnosis and treatment prevent you from really 'seeing' the patient in your office?
3 How do you experience the 'art' of medical practice?

# Closing the visit

◆ *Safe* (Julianne Moore). This is a perplexing film about Carol (Julianne Moore), a woman with unexplained physical symptoms who increasingly believes that she is being harmed by chemicals in the environment.

a (0:23:07–0:24:21). In this clip, Carol consults her primary care physician about her vague symptoms.

1 How well does this physician close the interview? Specifically, how well does he check for patient understanding, elicit questions about recommendations and provide appropriate education?

2   What are your reactions to the timing of the physician's question about illicit drug use?
3   What are some effective ways of closing a patient visit that is becoming too drawn out?

## Behavioral health referral

◆ *Safe* (Julianne Moore). See previous section on closing the visit for movie description.

a (0:32:48–0:34:08). In this scene, Carol and her husband are given a referral to a psychiatrist after being pronounced physically healthy.

1   How well does the physician explain his referral to a psychiatrist?
2   What is it about behavioral referrals that makes them particularly challenging?
3   What are some ways of successfully making a referral to a behavioral specialist?

## Dealing with awkward moments

◆ *Dr T and the Women* (Richard Gere). Dr T (Richard Gere) is a beloved obstetrician–gynecologist in Houston, Texas, who has an overly thriving solo practice.

a (0:00:00–0:01:45). In this clip, Dr T is performing a Pap smear and pelvic examination.

1   What is the overall 'feel' of this scene?
2   How do you juggle a medical examination with social niceties?
3   What strategies can physicians employ to make unpleasant physical examinations more comfortable for patients and themselves?
4   How do you prevent patients from possibly misinterpreting empathy offered during intimate examinations?

## Interruptions

◆ *Austin Powers* (Mike Myers, Elizabeth Hurley). This is a comedy about the perennial struggle between good, as embodied by Austin Powers (Mike Myers), and bad, as embodied by Dr Evil (also played by Mike Myers).

a (1:05:50–1:06:20). In this scene, Dr Evil interrupts his teenage son ad nauseam.

1   Obviously none of you interrupt at the level shown in this scene. However, studies *do* show that physicians often interrupt patients' initial statements. What is the impact of being interrupted?
2   What methods can you use to avoid interrupting, at least during patients' initial statements?

## References

1.  Stewart M. Effective physician–patient communication and health outcomes: a review. *Can Med Assoc J* 1995; **152**: 1423–33.
2.  Levinson W, Roter DL, Mullooly FP. Physician-patient communication: the relationship with malpractice claims among primary care physicians and surgeons. *JAMA* 1997; **277**: 553–9.
3.  Lipkin M, Putnam S, Lazare A. *The Medical Interview: clinical care, education and research.* New York: Springer-Verlag, 1995.
4.  Simpson M, Buckman R, Stewart M. Doctor–patient communication: the Toronto Consensus Statement. *BMJ* 1991; **303**: 1385–7.
5.  Makoul G. Essential elements of communication in medical encounters: the Kalamazoo Consensus Statement. *Acad Med* 2001; **76**: 390–3.

Chapter 18

# The professional and personal self of the physician

*Sam P Hooper Jr, Matthew Alexander, Terry A Allbright, Christine Wan, James K Burks and Patricia Lenahan*

Medical education traditionally guides the physician towards development of the professional self, often at the expense of the personal self. While biomedical approaches to medical education may not overtly impede development of the personal self, the lack of explicit attention to this domain fosters neglect and subtle devaluing of the personal self. Failing to pay attention to the importance of balance between personal and professional life sets the stage for problems in a variety of areas, including ethical behavior, relational dynamics, medical systems, physician–patient culture and physician impairment. Through the ongoing practice of self-reflection, the student and the practicing physician can explore issues that directly affect both their professional and personal self, making meaningful change possible. Film provides one avenue for fostering such reflection.

## Medical education

◆ *Patch Adams* (Robin Williams). This sentimental film is based on the true story of Hunter Adams (Robin Williams), a physician in West Virginia. He identifies his passion for helping people while he is an inpatient in a psychiatric hospital, and he decides to pursue medical school. While there, his provocative behaviors challenge the traditional system. Patch starts a free clinic and alternative hospital with other like-minded students.

a (0:18:01–0:19:28). In this scene, the Dean is addressing the incoming class of medical students. We hear him say that it is irrational to trust a human being. He concludes that 'It is our mission here to rigorously and ruthlessly train your humanity out of you and make you into something better. We're going to make doctors out of you.' He is spontaneously applauded by the medical faculty and students.

1 Does this scene bring back memories of your experiences in medical school? What were the expectations of medical training in your program and how were they communicated?
2 Do you believe that medical training enhances human potential or diminishes humanistic qualities? Did your medical training emphasize personal as well as professional development? What kinds of people were your mentors? What personal and professional attributes did they embody?

◆ *Wit* (Emma Thompson, Christopher Lloyd). This movie tells the story of Vivian Bearing (Emma Thompson), a 'force' in the field of English literature, whose academic specialty (the metaphysical poetry of John Donne) offers her a way to give meaning to her academic career and, now, to the indignities of her cancer treatment. The film illuminates Vivian's eloquent and deeply moving struggle for dignity, meaning and peace as she faces death.

a (0:31:00–0:35:00). This scene begins with Dr Bearing talking to the viewer about 'the most interesting aspects of my tenure as an inpatient.' As Dr Bearing lies in her hospital bed, she invites us to observe 'grand rounds.'

1  This scene powerfully demonstrates what is often valued in medical education by some attendings. What kind of information does Dr Kilekian (Christopher Lloyd) ask for? What responses gain his praise and provoke his criticism? Would Dr Kilekian have been a respected attending in your medical school? Would Jason have been a respected student?
2  When a diagnosis of depression is floated and 'shot down' by Jason, a female colleague asks him to ask the patient directly whether she is depressed. Why does the director give her, rather than one of her male colleagues, this task? In your training, were male and female students expected to attend to different aspects of medical care?

◆ *The Doctor* (William Hurt, Christine Lahti, Wendy Crewson). This movie is based on the book *A Taste of My Own Medicine*, by Ed Rosenbaum, MD. It is the story of Dr Jack McKee (William Hurt), a cardiopulmonary surgeon who, after receiving a diagnosis of laryngeal cancer, experiences being a patient himself. Through the course of the movie, Dr McKee's experience as a patient profoundly changes both his professional and personal self.

a (1:53:57–1:56:51). In this scene, Dr McKee informs his residents that they will be spending the next 72 hours as inpatients in the hospital. Dr McKee wants his residents to experience at first hand the trials and tribulations of being a patient so that they can emerge as more sensitive physicians.

1  Is it necessary for healthcare providers to actually *live* patient experiences in order to be empathic and helpful? For example, is it necessary for single residents to be married with children in order to provide effective counseling to parents?
2  Have you ever had a direct experiential educational experience (e.g. attending an AA meeting or being a patient in the hospital)? How did this compare with more didactic approaches to learning?
3  Are both types of experience equally instructive for the development of the personal and professional self?

## Physician–patient interactions

◆ *Wit* (Emma Thompson, Christopher Lloyd). See previous section on medical education for movie description.

a (0:14:13–0:23:44). As this scene begins, we see Dr Bearing being wheeled into the examination room by Susie, her nurse, where she meets Dr Jason Posner, a former student of hers who is now a Fellow in Oncology. We learn that Dr Posner took Dr Bearing's course in order to improve his prospects of medical school admission by 'appearing well-rounded.'

1 What is your evaluation of Dr Posner's medical interview and examination? If you were the doctor, would you do anything differently?
2 Was being 'well-rounded' important to your medical school admission? What does being 'well-rounded' mean to you now?

### Additional scene

a (1:00:00–1:11:10). For contrast, note the scene where Dr Bearing occludes her IV line in order to bring her nurse into the room. Susie, a nurturing, attentive nurse, eats a Popsicle with Dr Bearing and talks with her about her code status.

## Professional behavior

◆ *The Doctor* (William Hurt, Christine Lahti, Wendy Crewson). See earlier section on medical education for movie description.

a (0:01:00–0:05:11). In this opening scene there are some inappropriate physician behaviors taking place in the operating room. Dr McKee asks Nancy, the nurse, when she is going to run away with him. Then, during the surgery, while responding to a cardiac emergency, he tells her that he 'always trembles when she is near.' Dr McKee's favorite surgery-closing music begins to play. He and his other male colleagues sing along to the sexually explicit lyrics and try to coax Nancy into singing with them, but she refuses.

1 How would you rate the behaviors of Dr McKee and his colleagues in the surgery room in terms of professionalism?
2 What is the problem with these interactions? How comfortable did the nurse appear? How would you feel if you were in the operating room and these comments were made? Do they constitute harassment?
3 Would you take any action if these comments were made by a resident colleague?

## Hospital bureaucracy and patient–physician satisfaction

◆ *The Doctor* (William Hurt, Christine Lahti, Wendy Crewson). See earlier section on medical education for movie description.

a (0:28:16–0:32:14). In this scene, Dr McKee makes his first visit to the out-patient clinic for cancer treatment. During the process, he becomes enraged at the impersonal treatment that he receives within the medical system.

1 In what ways does your work setting diminish or enhance patient satisfaction? In what ways does it diminish or enhance physician satisfaction? Are the values usually found in one's personal life applicable to one's professional life?

2   In what ways can you empower your patients to best negotiate the hospital and/or clinic environment?
3   How can physicians effect change in their hospital or clinic environment?

## The impaired physician/work addiction

◆ *Drunks* (Richard Lewis, Dianne Wiest). This is a film that provides an in-depth look at the 12-step recovery process. It depicts an ethnically and socially diverse group of individuals who share their stories during an AA meeting. Each participant tells the group something about themselves and their ongoing daily struggle with sobriety.

a   (0:50:23–0:55:51). During the AA meeting, Rachel (Dianne Wiest) describes stealing Demerol from her patients, the loss of her husband, children and home, her entry into rehabilitation and her reinstatement as a physician by her hospital. Since becoming sober, she has been coming to AA only after realizing that her work addiction parallels her drug addiction. She realizes that she has not dealt with the source of her addictions.

1   How do you think an imbalance in Rachel's life led to her first using Demerol? Is her life still out of balance?
2   Physicians sometimes joke about being 'married or addicted' to their work. What do you think this means? What aspects of the physician lifestyle pose a risk for the development of chemical dependency? What constitutes a healthy relationship with one's work?
3   Has physician impairment been discussed in your training program? What are the signs and symptoms of impairment? How could you best approach a colleague whom you suspect shows signs of impairment?
4   What are the distinctions between *chemical* and *process* addictions? Name some other common process addictions.

## Legal issues in medicine

◆ *The Doctor* (William Hurt, Christine Lahti, Wendy Crewson). See earlier section on medical education for movie description.

a   (1:33:09–1:34:44). Dr McKee tells his partner that he will not testify in court to corroborate his partner's care of a litigious patient. Dr McKee says that he has to be truthful about the patient's medical history. His partner says they have always 'covered' for each other, and is taken aback by Dr McKee's decision.

1   What do you think of Dr McKee's decision not to cover for his colleague?
2   How would you respond to a colleague's request for you to testify about the care that he or she provided, when you knew that a deliberate effort had been made to omit the full story or when an error had occurred? What consequences might you face if you testified? What consequences might you face if you decided *not* to testify?
3   Do you think Dr Kaplan is asking Dr McKee to help him as a friend or as a colleague? In a similar situation, how would you reconcile your loyalty to a colleague with your legal and ethical responsibility to tell the truth?

4   How has your practice changed because of concerns over litigation?
5   What are your concerns about malpractice issues? Are they professional or personal?
6   Are there other issues that might require a difficult dialogue with colleagues? What are the best ways to handle such discussions?

## The medical marriage and family

◆ *The Doctor* (William Hurt, Christine Lahti, Wendy Crewson). See earlier section on medical education for movie description.

a   (0:23:52–0:24:43). In this scene, Dr Jack McKee returns home after receiving the news that he has a laryngeal tumor. Neither he nor his wife, Ann (Christine Lahti), expects the other to be home. Ann makes an effort to be enthusiastic about 'a night together' when she learns of Jack's plan to stay at home with his family. Ann calls to their son, Nicky, and tells him to say 'hi' to his father. Nicky picks up the phone, thinking that his father is still at work. With a fanfare, Ann announces that Jack is actually at home. When Nicky realizes this, he waves to his father and then runs off to play.

1   In this vignette, we are shown a stereotypical medical marriage and family. How well do you think Jack and Ann have balanced their personal and professional lives? Speculate about how this family functions. When Jack and Ann married, do you think they agreed to be married in this way? As you think about Jack and Ann's relationship, does this change how you think about the medical marriage?
2   When Nicky picks up the phone, what does this tell you about the relationship between Jack and his son? Do you think that Jack anticipated having this kind of relationship with his son? How do you think it happened? What do you think the consequences are for both of them?
3   Does this scene bring to mind ways in which patients either involve or disengage themselves from their partners during the course of an illness? How can you assist patients and their families in having open discussions about serious illness?

b   (1:35:00–1:35:57). At the hospital, Jack and Ann reflect on their lack of communication. Information about dinner dates and appointments is often communicated by Jack's secretary.

1   Do you think that this is a common pattern in medical marriages?
2   What potential problems might arise for couples with such limited opportunities for communication? How might such a pattern be changed?

## Gender and medicine

◆ *The Doctor* (William Hurt, Christine Lahti, Wendy Crewson). See earlier section on medical education for movie description.

a   (00:20:03–00:23:47). In this scene, Dr McKee is evaluated by Dr Leslie Abbott (Wendy Crewson), a throat surgeon. Dr Abbott is brusque, impersonal, and insensitive to the emotional aspects of Dr McKee's examination and diagnosis.

1 Do you believe that the public has different expectations for female physicians than those it has for male physicians? Does the public behave differently with female physicians and male physicians? If so, how?
2 As a physician, have you ever felt *harassed* by opposite-sex patients? If so, how have you handled this?
3 Is there a place for stereotypically 'feminine' values in medicine (e.g. cooperation, empathy, nurturance and emotional responsiveness)?

◆ *Patch Adams* (Robin Williams). See earlier section on medical education for movie description.

a (0:34:13–0:35:18). In this scene, a medical student describes the pressures that she feels as a minority female.

1 How applicable is this personal account to today's medical school environment?
2 What pressures, if any, have you experienced as a women in the medical field?

# Chapter 19

# The difficult patient

*Matthew Alexander and Jay C Williams*

A landmark article by James Groves described four distinct types of 'hateful' patient, namely the 'dependent clinger,' the 'entitled demander,' the 'manipulative help rejecter' and the 'self-destructive denier.'[1] 'Hateful' patients, while obviously not deserving of hate, are *difficult* in that they evoke a variety of negative feelings in caregivers. If properly handled, such feelings can lead to insight and exemplary patient care.[2,3] However, if poorly handled, these feelings can compromise care and wreak havoc on the professional and personal life of the healthcare provider. Groves' article provides a typology for classification of difficult patients to which clinicians can easily relate, normalizes the negative feelings engendered by these patients and offers appropriate coping strategies for managing them.

As might be expected, there is considerable overlap between Groves' four types of 'hateful' patient and several classic personality disorders, most notably paranoid (cluster A), borderline and narcissistic (cluster B), and dependent (cluster C) personality disorder.[4] In addition, difficult patients such as those with substance abuse problems, depression, anxiety, bipolar disease and schizophrenia may also evoke strongly negative feelings in the provider. Clips illustrating these diagnostic categories can be found in other sections.

## Dependent clingers

Dependent clingers are those patients with a seemingly bottomless need for care. They tend to evoke aversion. They fall into two general categories, one overlapping with the diagnosis of dependent personality disorder and the other overlapping with the diagnosis of borderline personality disorder.

◆ *What About Bob?* (Bill Murray, Richard Dreyfuss). This 'dark' but very funny movie tells the story of Bob Wiley (Bill Murray), a highly anxious individual who invades the personal life of his therapist, Dr Leo Marvin (Richard Dreyfuss).

a (0:07:11–0:11:40). Bob uses flattery to manipulate and 'hook' Dr Marvin into taking him on as a patient.

b (0:23:50–0:26:20). In this clip, Bob shows up uninvited at Dr Marvin's summer village where he and his family are on vacation, and he proceeds to flagrantly demonstrate his extreme dependency needs.

1　What type of personality disorder is Bob most likely to have?
2　What types of feelings does Bob evoke in Dr Marvin? What feelings are evoked in you as you observe this clip?

3  How does Dr Marvin attempt to manage his negative feelings? How successful is he? How does he attempt to set appropriate boundaries with Bob? How successful is he?
4  Have you ever had your personal boundaries violated by a dependent patient? What feelings were evoked in you? How did you handle the situation?
5  What are some of the best ways to manage an overly dependent patient?

◆ *Fatal Attraction* (Michael Douglas, Glenn Close). This film tells the story of a romantic involvement between married attorney Dan Gallagher (Michael Douglas) and Alex Forrest (Glenn Close). When Dan tries to end the affair, Alex responds with frantic efforts to prevent him from doing so.

a  (0:31:00–0:37:00). When Dan attempts to leave Alex and return home after a weekend tryst, she responds with rage and a suicidal gesture.

1  What elements of borderline personality disorder does this clip reveal?
2  What feelings are evoked in Dan during this clip? What feelings are evoked in you as you watch the clip?
3  Have you ever had a patient with borderline personality disorder in your practice? Have you ever known a borderline individual in your personal life? What were these individuals like? How would you distinguish between a person with borderline personality disorder and borderline traits? What is the origin of borderline personality disorder (e.g. genetic, environmental)?
4  What is the best way to manage borderline patients?

## Entitled demanders

Entitled demanders use intimidation rather than flattery as a way to manipulate others. They tend to evoke fear and counter-attack in clinicians. There is an overlap between this 'type' and narcissistic personality disorder with its 'pattern of grandiosity, need for admiration and lack of empathy' (DSM-IV-TR). Often underlying such patients' sense of entitlement is a low self-esteem.

◆ *Analyze This* (Robert De Niro, Billy Crystal). This is a hilarious movie about a powerful crime racketeer, Paul Vitti (Robert De Niro), with panic disorder, and his reluctant therapist, Ben Sobel (Billy Crystal).

a  (0:16:28–0:22:55). In this scene, Vitti interrupts a session-in-progress to demand that Dr Sobel take him on as a patient.

1  How does Dr Sobel respond to Vitti's demands? What feelings are evoked in you as you watch this scene?
2  Have you ever had an 'entitled demander' in your practice? What are the best ways to handle difficult encounters with such patients?

◆ *As Good As It Gets* (Jack Nicholson, Helen Hunt). This film documents the relationship between Melvin Udall (Jack Nicholson), an obsessive-compulsive novelist, and Carol Conelly (Helen Hunt), a good-hearted waitress.

a  (0:40:34–0:42:09). In this scene, Udall barges into his former therapist's office.

1  How does Udall attempt to get the therapist to see him?

2 How does the therapist respond? What would have happened if the therapist became upset by Udall's provocations?

## Manipulative help rejectors

'Manipulative help rejectors' use their symptoms as a 'ticket of admission' to the healthcare professional's office and then proceed to reject all interventions. They tend to evoke guilt and inadequacy in caregivers. There may be some overlap between this 'type' and paranoid personality disorder, antisocial personality disorder and somatization disorder.

◆ *The Odd Couple* (Jack Lemmon, Walter Matthau). This is an endearing movie about Felix (Jack Lemmon), who is an obsessive-compulsive complainer, and Oscar (Walter Matthau), his messy but supportive friend.

a (0:34:10–0:38:10). In this scene, Felix and Oscar walk to and then sit down in a restaurant, where Felix talks about his marital problems and attempts to 'clear his sinuses.'

1 What are some possible underlying motivations for Felix's physical complaints?
2 What are the responses of Oscar (and the other customers) to Felix's somatic complaints? How receptive is Felix to his friend's advice? How are these interpersonal dynamics similar to those between healthcare providers and manipulative help rejectors?
3 What is the relationship between Oscar's life stress and the onset of his sinus symptoms? How receptive are help rejectors to having healthcare providers make an explicit link between their somatic complaints and underlying psychological stress?
4 What are the optimal ways of handling manipulative help rejectors in clinical practice?

## Self-destructive deniers

'Self-destructive deniers' unconsciously wish to end their lives. Like the other three types of 'hateful' patient, they too are profoundly dependent, but they evoke all of the previously mentioned negative emotions in caregivers *plus* a wish that such patients would just die and 'get it over with.' There is some overlap between this 'type' and individuals with antisocial, borderline and histrionic personality disorder.

◆ *Leaving Las Vegas* (Nicholas Cage, Elisabeth Shue). This very dark movie tells the story of an end-stage alcoholic, Vin Sanderson (Nicholas Cage), and Sera (Elisabeth Shue), a prostitute with a heart of gold. Despite Sera's best efforts, Vin dies from chronic, unremitting alcohol abuse.

a (1:22:12–1:26:47). In this scene, Vin awakens in a cold sweat and immediately consumes two bottles of vodka. Sera unsuccessfully attempts to steer him towards seeking medical help.

1 What feelings are evoked in Sera by Vin? What feelings are evoked in you as you watch this scene?
2 Have you ever dealt with severely self-destructive patients while doing inpatient services? What have been some inappropriate ways in which these patients have been handled?
3 What is the best way to manage the 'self-destructive denier' in clinical practice?

## References

1. Groves J. Taking care of the hateful patient. *NEJM* 1978; **298**: 883–7.
2. Zinn W. Doctors have feelings too. *JAMA* 1988; **259**: 3296–8.
3. Gorlin R, Zucker H. Physicians' reactions to patients. *NEJM* 1983; **308**: 1059–63.
4. DeLong D, Smith G, Grange J. Does that difficult patient have a personality disorder? *Emerg Med* 1996; December: 75–96.

# Chapter 20

# Ethics and human values

*Pablo Gonzalez Blasco and Matthew Alexander*

In ancient times, education in ethics and human values was reinforced through the art of storytelling.[1] Storytelling represents a solution to the educational problem caused by the fact that most individuals, especially young people such as medical students and residents, have only been exposed to a limited range of life experience. Storytelling, whether it be through theater, literature, opera or cinema, has the capacity to supplement young learners' understanding of ethics and human values by exposing them to people and situations they have not yet encountered.

Engaging learners emotionally and promoting reflection in them are other essential elements in promoting a meaningful discussion of values and ethics.[2] In our experience, cinema, arguably our most popular current medium for story-telling, provides an outstanding resource in this regard.

The importance of values and ethics in medical education is clear. Given the ever-emerging technologies that preoccupy medical learners, there is a compelling need to reinforce, inspire and educate future healthcare professionals about the human dimension of their work. Otherwise our students and residents run the risk of becoming mechanics rather than healthcare providers. Issues of values and ethics are central to any attempt to foster humanism in medical learners.

In his use of cinemeducation to teach humanism to medical students, Dr Blasco makes comments while the movie clips are showing.[3,4] Because students are involved in their own reflective process, they may at times disagree with the teacher's comments and reach their own conclusions. Talking during a film clip may work best with films that have subtitles.

The film clips suggested in this chapter are also useful when attempting to inspire and motivate young learners. Part of their power lies in the fact that they do not deal directly with medicine.

## Vocation for doctoring

◆ *The Bone Collector* (Denzel Washington, Angelina Jolie). This film tells the story of Lincoln Rhyme (Denzel Washington), a seasoned homicide investigator who, because of a tragic accident that incapacitates him, must team up with a young rookie, Amelia Donaghy (Angelina Jolie), in order to hunt a serial killer.

a (0:59:44–1:02:15). In this scene, Rhyme attempts to persuade Amelia not to give up on her dream of being a detective.

1  What gifts do you bring to medicine?
2  How can you best develop these gifts?

3  Have you ever thought about leaving medicine? If so, why? What caused you to stay?

◆ *Patch Adams* (Robin Williams). This is a movie about Dr Hunter 'Patch' Adams and his experiences during medical school. Despite the emphasis on objectivity in medical culture, Patch tries to bring warmth and healing to his interactions with patients, challenging the status quo by interacting with patients in unconventional ways.

a  (0:32:26–0:35:18). In this scene, Patch disrupts his medical school study group by asking provocative questions about medicine.

1  What do you remember about your decision to become a physician?
2  Why *do* you want to be a doctor? Have your motivations changed over the years?
3  What memories (good or bad) of medical school are evoked by this clip?

## Keeping your idealism

◆ *Tucker: the Man and his Dream* (Jeff Bridges, Joan Allen, Martin Landau). This movie is based on the real life of Preston Tucker (Jeff Bridges), who built and attempted to market a sleek new automobile in 1948. It is a film about the American dream and the power of corporations to successfully defeat competition.

a  (01:43:20–01:44:20). In this scene, we witness Tucker's adaptive response to being acquitted by a jury but still denied the right to build any more of his automobiles. Despite only having been able to build 50 cars before being stopped by the Big Three automobile manufacturers, Tucker still feels victorious.

1  What level of idealism do you bring to medicine?
2  What have been the challenges to maintaining your idealism?
3  Have you been able to maintain your idealism? If not, what has replaced it?

◆ *October Sky* (Jake Gyllenhaal, Chris Cooper, Laura Dern). Set in the 1950s, this film tells the story of a group of boys from a coal-mining town who become fascinated with rocketry and space exploration, despite the reservations of their parents. The movie centers on how this particular conflict plays out between Homer (Jake Gyllenhaal) and his coal-mining father (Chris Cooper).

a  (01:17:31–01:20:30, 01:35:14–01:39:50). In these scenes, Homer differentiates himself psychologically from his father. Despite his father's admonitions, Homer refuses to go back to coal mining and clings to his dream of building a rocket.

1  What types of family challenge have you faced in making your own dreams come true?
2  How can you help your patients to persevere in the face of multiple challenges?

## Facing difficulties

◆ *The Truman Show* (Jim Carrey, Ed Harris, Laura Linney). This movie is about 'reality television' before it became such a mainstay of our culture. Truman (Jim Carrey) is an ordinary man whose every move is televised and broadcast to the nation without his knowledge.

a (01:24:07–01:29:03). In this scene, the director of the Truman Show (Ed Harris) attempts to drown Truman in front of a live audience by capsizing his boat. Truman, who now realizes that his life is being televised, attempts to sail to freedom by tying himself to the mast of his boat, and miraculously survives.

1   What does this scene teach you about perseverance?
2   What difficulties have you overcome in your life?
3   Have there been times in your medical career when you felt like giving up? What helped you to survive?

## Understanding suffering and pain

◆ *Shadowlands* (Anthony Hopkins, Debra Winger). This movie tells the true story of CS Lewis (Anthony Hopkins), an acclaimed author and professor, and his relationship with Joy Gresham (Debra Winger), a spirited divorcee from New York. During the course of their relationship, Lewis confronts the joy and pain of loving deeply.

a (0:10:17–0:11:58). CS Lewis addresses a church congregation about the topic of suffering.

1   What is CS Lewis's perspective on the role of suffering in life? What is your perspective?
2   How have you been able to cope with the suffering that you observe as a healthcare professional? What has been the most difficult clinical case for you in this regard? What made this particular case so difficult?
3   How have you been able to help patients and their families to cope with the pain and suffering that result from medical conditions?

b (01:45:50–01:48:11). In this scene, Joy Gresham and CS Lewis have an intimate discussion about Joy's impending death from Ewing's sarcoma, a type of bone cancer.

1   What is Gresham's philosophy of suffering? How does her philosophy correspond to your own?
2   What lessons do you take from this scene?
3   Why is it so hard for people to talk about death? In what ways can you facilitate such discussions within families?

◆ *The Spitfire Grill* (Ellen Burstyn, Marcia Gay Harden, Will Patton, Alison Elliot). This is a movie about redemption in a young woman who relocates to Gilead, Maine, after being in prison for the past five years.

a (01:31:36–01:35:05). In this scene, Percy Talbot (Alison Elliot) tells her story of a previous rape and subsequent miscarriage to a friend. Percy's friend listens quietly to her story and then places her hand on Percy's shoulder without saying a word.

1 Why does listening in and of itself help to reduce suffering?
2 How can you be a better listener in the midst of a busy practice?
3 What are the best ways to encourage patients to talk about difficult aspects of their life?

# Transcendence

◆ *Marvin's Room* (Meryl Streep, Leonardo DiCaprio, Diane Keaton, Robert De Niro, Hume Cronyn). This powerful family drama tells the story of two sisters, independent Lee (Meryl Streep) and kind-hearted Bessie (Diane Keaton), who are taking care of their chronically ill father, Marvin (Hume Cronyn).

a (01:26:53–01:28:02). In this emotional scene, Bessie, who has leukemia and is searching for a bone-marrow donor, tells Lee how grateful she is that she has been able to care for their father. She deeply affects her more cynical sister by directly stating her feelings about selflessness.

1 How does the act of service to others allow us to transcend mortal limits?
2 How are you able to demonstrate 'love' in your clinical work?

◆ *Dead Man Walking* (Susan Sarandon, Sean Penn). This movie tells the story of the close involvement of a nun, Sister Helen (Susan Sarandon), with a convicted murderer, Matthew (Sean Penn), who is awaiting execution.

a (1:36:00–1:37:30). In these scenes, Sister Helen is ministering to Matthew before his imminent execution.

1 What do these scenes tell us about the transformative power of love?
2 How do you understand the common occurrence of 'jail-house conversions'?

## References

1. MacIntyre A. *Tras la Virtud (After the Virtue)*. Barcelona: Crítica, 1987.
2. Retegui AR. *Pulchrum*. Madrid: Rialp, 1999.
3. Blasco PG. *Medicina de Familia e Cinema: recursos humanisticos na Educacão Médica*. São Paulo: Casa do Psicologo, 2002.
4. Blasco PG. Literature and movies for medical students. *Fam Med* 2001; **33**: 426–8.

# Chapter 21

# Medical error

*Ruth Hart*

Since the publication in 1999 of the Institute of Medicine report entitled *To Err is Human* and the follow-up report entitled *Crossing the Bridges*, the topic of medical error has moved from the realm of concealment, shame and guilt to one of analysis, open discussion and prevention. In an effort to promote a 'culture of safety,' film clips will be recommended that highlight necessary areas of reflection on this sensitive topic that is pertinent to healthcare providers.

## Medical error: the price to be paid

◆ *The Verdict* (James Mason, Paul Newman, Charlotte Rampling). This is a movie about Frank Galvin (Paul Newman), a down-and-out alcoholic Boston attorney given a 'sure-win' medical practice case. The case concerns an alleged medical mistake made during a delivery which left the mother in a vegetative state. The key piece of information needed to disclose the cover-up promulgated by the acclaimed specialist is provided by tracking down the nurse who witnessed the error and has since left the profession.

a (1:47:20–1:56:47). The trial scene shows the collision between the medical and legal professions. We see the importance of detailed medical records in resolving cases of medical negligence, and are confronted with ethical issues related to falsification of medical charts and the cover-up of medical error. Other issues, such as professional loyalty, personal gain, personal cost of medical mistakes, monetary compensation for lost quality of life and intimidation by the specialist, also surface in this scene.

1 What steps should you take if you witness a medical mistake or are asked to cover one up?
2 What are the potential personal costs (e.g. mental, professional, etc.) of witnessing a medical error as opposed to committing a medical error? Are they the same?
3 What are the reasons for intimidation in medical practice and medical education? What is the effect on the intimidator and on the person who is being intimidated?

## Errors in judgement

◆ *Frankenstein* (Kenneth Branagh, Helena Bonham Carter, Robert De Niro). Kenneth Branagh's film version of Mary Shelley's classic monster tale tells the story of Dr Victor Frankenstein (Kenneth Branagh) and his obsessive quest for knowledge at all costs, and the disastrous consequences of his actions.

a (0:45:43–0:50:20). In this clip, the half-crazed Dr Frankenstein attempts to give the spark of life to his inanimate creation. The object of his obsession takes on a living form (Robert De Niro) and, to Frankenstein's horror, is hideous and turns on him with tremendous destructive power.

1 What are some occasions during the training and career of physicians when the intensity of their focus can lead them to lose perspective and make errors of judgement?
2 Dr Frankenstein's obsession with creating life causes him to ignore the consequences of his actions. Consider examples of circumstances when obvious harmful consequences were not taken into account in medical decision making (e.g. Tuskegee experiment, cloning).
3 Mary Shelley suggests that a serious danger exists when people allow their work to alienate them from whom and what they love in life. What other danger signals should a physician look for in order to avoid becoming alienated? How do we stay balanced in our approach to work?

## Communicating about error

◆ *The Citadel* (Robert Donat, Rex Harrison, Rosalind Russell, Ralph Richardson). Based on the novel written by the physician AJ Cronin, this movie is set in the 1920s and tells the story of Andrew Manson (Robert Donat), an enthusiastic young Scottish doctor. Dr Manson moves from a Welsh mining town to London after being tempted to pursue money and prestige, but soon returns to his ideals after experiencing a series of moral and ethical dilemmas.

a (0:01:34–0:01:41). In this selection of scenes, Dr Manson is visited by his friend and former colleague Denny (Ralph Richardson), who rebukes him for his fascination with fame and prosperity. Denny is critically injured, and Dr Manson calls upon a surgeon of supposedly high repute to save his life, only to see at first hand that this specialist is a quack. The death of his friend after surgery forces Manson to confront the surgeon who committed the gross error that led to his friend's death. He must also confront his own false ideals.

1 What feelings and reactions do physicians experience when they are involved in a medical error? To whom can they turn at this time?
2 What difficulties would you face if you witnessed a medical error made by a colleague?
3 What are the universal elements of this scenario that make this clip, over 50 years later, still relevant to physicians today?

# Chapter 22

# Lifestyle modification

*Patricia Lenahan, Anna Pavlov and Matthew Alexander*

The USA has witnessed a dramatic increase in the number of individuals who are overweight, suffer from diabetes, or who engage in other behaviorally risky behaviors such as smoking and drinking. Consequently, preventive care, lifestyle modification and anticipatory guidance are areas in which family physicians have an opportunity to make a great impact on the lives of their patients and their families. This chapter addresses some of the more common addictive behaviors in our society, and illustrates a variety of behavioral and motivational approaches to lifestyle modification.

## Smoking cessation/nicotine addiction

◆ *Cat's Eye* (Drew Barrymore, James Woods, Alan King, Robert Hays). This film consists of three suspense and horror tales based on stories by Stephen King. The three stories are bound together by a cat. The first story involves Dick Morrison (James Woods), who tries to quit smoking by going to Quitters Inc, a smoking cessation program run by mobster Mr Tonatti (Alan King), who gives new meaning to the term *aversion therapy.*

a (0:07:29–0:10:12). In this scene, Dick Morrison meets Quitters Inc counselor Mr Tonatti, who explains that being available to clients is only part of the program. Mr Tonatti knows about Dick's family, talks about recidivism rates and demonstrates aversion therapy with the cat.

1   How successful is aversion therapy in achieving abstinence?
2   What other types of treatment should be considered?
3   What approach would you consider?
4   How would you assess the patient's current motivation for treatment?

b (0:13:15–0:14:33). Dick is at home and spills a drink. His wife asks what is wrong and Dick tells her that he has quit smoking. She responds by saying 'When? Five minutes ago? Dick replies 'Six hours and 23 minutes.' His wife says that even if he does not succeed both she and their daughter are grateful to him for trying.

1   What role does family support play in supporting or curtailing addictive behaviors?
2   What effect can a spouse's lack of confidence have on a patient who is trying to quit?
3   How would you respond to a patient who tells you the exact number of hours and minutes he has been smoke-free? How could you encourage such a patient to continue his program?

c (0:22:45–0:25:22). This is a rather surreal scene in which Dick and his wife attend a party. The party is seen from Dick's perspective, in which everyone is smoking. He begins to see people with cigarettes in their ears and children smoking. Dick has been smoke-free for two weeks now.

1 What does this scene portray about the impact of quitting smoking?
2 What recommendations would you make to a patient who associates social activities with smoking?

d (0:25:48–0:27:36). Dick is caught in a traffic jam and is becoming more and more agitated. He rummages through the glove box and finds an old packet of cigarettes. He begins chewing gum, but keeps looking at the cigarettes. Eventually he lights up and begins smoking.

1 What situations or behaviors can predispose a patient to relapse?
2 How can patients be assisted in dealing with relapse situations?
3 What is the impact of substituting gum chewing for smoking? Is this a successful approach to smoking cessation?

e (0:33:13–0:33:58). Dick is weighing in at Quitters Inc. Mr Tonatti tells him that he has gained eight pounds in six months, and gives him diet pills.

1 How would you approach a patient who is substituting eating for smoking?
2 How would you address a patient's concerns that they will gain weight if they quit smoking?
3 Would you give diet pills to a patient who engages in addictive behaviors?

## Dieting and weight loss

◆ *I Don't Buy Kisses Anymore* (Jason Alexander, Lainie Kazan, Nia Peeples, Eileen Brennan). Bernie Fisbine (Jason Alexander) is an overweight man in his thirties who runs the family shoe store and lives with his mother (Lainie Kazan). Bernie is looking for a girlfriend when he meets Tress Garabaldi (Nia Peeples), a psychology student who thinks that Bernie will make a great subject for her thesis on overeating.

a (0:08:30–0:09:30). Bernie is sitting down to dinner with his mother. He places some meat on his plate, which his mother quickly removes. She tells him that if he loses 30 pounds like the doctor says, then he will be able to eat whatever he wants.

1 What is the role of the family in facilitating weight loss?
2 How helpful do you think Bernie's mother is in dealing with his weight problem?
3 Does her type of approach help or hinder patients?

b (0:43:33–0:44:50). Bernie was unsuccessful in getting a date with Tress and comes home. He immediately heads for the refrigerator and makes himself a sandwich.

c (0:46:50–0:47:25). Tress talks to a friend about her research and discusses how stress affects addicts.

1 What role does stress play in addictive behaviors?
2 How would you counsel patients about stress reduction and addictive behaviors?

d (0:57:30–0:58:29). Bernie is having dinner with Tress, who comments on how much he ate the other night. She talks with him about 'falling off the wagon.'

1 How would you describe Tress's behavior? Is she helpful or harmful to Bernie's weight-loss program?
2 How does Tress's talking about 'falling off the wagon' affect Bernie?
3 How would you discuss relapse with patients?
4 What anticipatory guidance would you offer to patients regarding relapse prevention?

♦ *Heavy* (Shelly Winters, Deborah Harry, Liv Tyler, Pruitt Taylor Vincent). Victor (Pruitt Taylor Vincent) is an overweight cook who lives with his domineering mother, Dolly (Shelly Winters), and works in her diner. Victor, a virgin, becomes attracted to the new waitress, Callie (Liv Tyler), and begins to fantasize about her, which frightens Dolly, who fears that she is losing control over her son.

a (0:49:53–0:50:44). Victor is in the grocery store. He picks up a can of 'light and fit' protein powder instead of the rich and fatty foods he had been looking at.

1 What factors are motivating Victor's desire to change?
2 As a physician, how can you motivate a patient to make healthy lifestyle modifications?
3 Where does Victor's behavior fit into the Stages of Change model?
4 How can you assess resistance to change?

# Exercise

♦ *I Don't Buy Kisses Anymore* (Jason Alexander, Lainie Kazan, Nia Peeples, Eileen Brennan). See previous section on dieting and weight loss for movie description.

a (0:24:08–0:29:24). Tress takes Bernie to the gym and introduces him to a personal trainer. This is Bernie's first visit to the gym, and the trainer takes him from a stationery bicycle to a treadmill, and then to the pool, where he is told to swim ten laps. Bernie arrives home late, barely able to walk. The next morning at breakfast his mother is trying to talk him out of going to the gym again. Bernie tells her that he will be going every day and that he will probably be worse when he gets home tonight.

1 How does 'overdoing' affect compliance with exercise prescriptions?
2 What is the role of the family or significant others in promoting behavior change?
3 How would you counsel patients who 'overdo' behavioral changes?

b (0:29:45–0:30:48). Bernie is at the gym lifting weights, working out on the life cycle and then walking on the treadmill as a young woman jogs next to him.

1 What effect does seeing other individuals who are more physically fit have on patients who have just initiated an exercise program?

## Diabetes management

◆ *Soul Food* (Vanessa Williams, Vivica A Fox, Nia Long, Brandon Hammond, Irma P Hall). This movie is the story of an extended family who share Sunday dinner, family values, traditions and secrets.

a (0:12:16–0:12:52). Big Mama (Irma P Hall) is cooking with her arm over one of the burners of the stove. She does not realize that she has burned her arm until her grandson shouts at her. Immediately her daughters begin to barrage her with questions about taking her insulin, seeing her doctor and caring for her diabetes. Big Mama replies that she does not need a doctor – she only needs her turpentine, salve and herbs.

1  How would you address this patient's understanding of her disease?
2  How would you assess Big Mama's motivation and resistance to following a diabetic regimen?
3  What is the role of the family in aiding or hindering patient compliance?
4  What is your understanding of this patient's values and perceptions about risky behaviors?
5  What direct interventions could be used to address patient compliance?

## Substance use

◆ *Drunks* (Richard Lewis, Faye Dunaway, Dianne Wiest). This film provides an in-depth look at the 12-step recovery process as it follows an ethnically and socially diverse group of individuals who share their stories during their weekly AA meetings.

a (0:20:48–0:22:20). Jim (Richard Lewis) passes by several bars and liquor stores after sharing his 'story' at an AA meeting. He buys a pint of bourbon, opens the bottle, smells the bourbon, caresses the bottle and finally leaves it behind.

1  How would you counsel a patient who related an episode such as this?
2  What are the risks of such a patient drinking again?
3  How would you assess the patient and counsel them against relapse?

b (0:26:20–0:27:30). Jim goes into another liquor store. The owner, Harry, refuses to sell him any alcohol, reminds him that he has been sober for two years and tells Jim that he will not get drunk from alcohol bought in this store.

1  What role does the liquor-store owner have in addressing Jim's sobriety?
2  What other actions might the store owner have taken?
3  What do you think is the likelihood that Jim will maintain his sobriety?
4  How would you counsel a patient like Jim?

c (0:30:10–0:30:53). Jim goes into another liquor store, purchases a fifth of bourbon and begins drinking.

1  What prompted this relapse?
2  What signs and behaviors might have contributed to the relapse?
3  What was the impact of sharing his story in AA on his current drinking?

**d** (1:05:35–1:08:35). A young woman attending the AA meeting raises her hand to speak. She says that she would rather be dead than sober. She says that she does not feel any better with AA, and that she drank alcohol and smoked a joint this morning so she could get through the day. She adds that she had planned to go out and get drunk tonight, but came to the meeting instead because she wants someone to stop her.

1   How would you describe this woman's level of understanding of her disease?
2   How would you help a patient who expresses similar feelings?
3   What could you do to enhance such a patient's motivation to achieve sobriety?

## Dual addictions

◆ *28 Days* (Sandra Bullock, Reni Santoni). Gwen (Sandra Bullock) ruins her sister's wedding after arriving drunk. She ends up in a 28-day inpatient program for alcoholics and addicts.

**a** (0:14:45–0:15:09). The group is on an outing and stops at a convenience store. Gwen asks for a packet of cigarettes and is told that they are out of stock. She becomes enraged and says that these people out here are addicts and they need their cigarettes like they need air. Finally she asks the store clerk if she has gum.

1   What is the impact of substituting one addictive behavior for another?
2   Which addiction would you treat first, nicotine or alcohol? Or, would you treat both behaviors at the same time?

## Anger management

◆ *Anger Management* (Jack Nicholson, Adam Sandler, Marisa Tomei). A marketing executive, Dave (Adam Sandler), is a mild-mannered individual who, through a series of comical, escalating misperceptions, is sentenced for assault and battery against a flight attendant. He is ordered to pay a fine and attend 20 hours of anger management training. His anger management coach, Dr Rydel (Jack Nicholson), goes overboard when monitoring his behavior, making the audience wonder why he himself has not been sentenced to treatment. A twist in the plot exposes the involvement of Dave's girlfriend (Marisa Tomei) in these bizarre events.

**a** (0:08:11–0:08:45). In court with his attorney, Dave is sentenced for assault and battery against a flight attendant on a recent flight. He is ordered to pay a fine and attend 20 hours of anger management training.

**b** (0:08:51–0:12:37). Dave shows up for his first anger management class. He recognizes the facilitator, Dr Rydel, as the passenger who sat next to him on the plane and who witnessed the misunderstanding which resulted in his assault and battery charge. Dave asks Dr Rydel to sign off for him because, despite the charge, he did not do anything wrong. Dr Rydel suggests that he should attend one class and then he will sign him off. The scene ends when Dr Rydel suggests that others in the class introduce themselves to Dave.

1 While the recommendation for anger management treatment may be court ordered, are there circumstances in which you might suggest anger management training to a patient?
2 What health conditions are associated with anger, hostility and other type A behavior?
3 How would you approach an angry patient in your practice?
4 What anger management resources are available in your community?

# Part V

## Specific populations

# Chapter 23

# Gay, lesbian, bisexual and transgender issues

*Anthony Zamudio*

Gay, lesbian, bisexual and transgender (GLBT) patients' sexual orientation, identity and lifestyle often remain invisible within the healthcare system. Fears of discrimination, persecution and compromised care contribute to the GLBT patient's avoidance of routine healthcare screening and delay in seeking treatment. GLBT patients are at risk for specific conditions, such as gastrointestinal infections, sexually transmitted diseases, breast and ovarian cancer, and endometrial and colon cancer. They are also at risk for depression, suicide, substance abuse, eating disorders, intimate partner abuse and victimization from hate crimes. These conditions often remain undetected and greatly impact on health.[1]

As gatekeepers to the healthcare system, family physicians play a significant role in addressing healthcare issues specific to GLBT patients. Knowledge of and ease with GLBT issues enable the family physician to conduct a more effective medical interview and help these patients to establish greater trust in the physician–patient relationship. This chapter reviews some of the developmental and psychosocial issues that can influence GLBT patients' presentation and medical management.

## Coming out

### Coming out to the self

◆ *Beautiful Thing* (Glen Berry, Scott Neal, Linda Henry). Jamie (Glen Berry) is a quiet boy who is frequently picked on at school. Ste (Scott Neal) is Jamie's classmate and a school athlete. Ste lives next door with his abusive father and older brother.

a (0:35:25–0:42:35). Ste is beaten by his brother and finds refuge in Jamie's home. As the two boys sleep side by side in bed, they discover their mutual sexual attraction.

1 How would you respond to an adolescent disclosing his or her confusion about homosexual feelings?
2 How comfortable are you about eliciting sexual histories from adolescents? What would you say to a teenager who told you he or she is gay or lesbian?

### Coming out to each other

◆ *Beautiful Thing* (Glen Berry, Scott Neal, Linda Henry). See previous section on coming out to the self for movie description.

a (0:44:05–0:48:22). As their homosexual feelings awaken, Jamie secretly seeks out gay reading material and Ste avoids Jamie. At a party, Jamie confronts Ste's avoidance and acknowledges his love for him.

1 How would you respond to a dependent minor who wants to 'come out' to their parents and close friends?
2 If a patient told you they were planning on 'coming out,' how would you assess whether they had fully considered the issues prior to disclosure? What issues need to be considered prior to disclosure of homosexuality? What advice might you give your patient?

## Coming out to a parent

◆ *Beautiful Thing* (Glen Berry, Scott Neal, Linda Henry). See earlier section on coming out to the self for movie description.

a (0:59:45–1:11:17). Jamie's mother, Sandra (Linda Henry), discovers her son's homosexuality and confronts him.

1 How equipped do you feel to respond to parents' concerns that their son/ daughter might be homosexual?
2 What resources are available in your community to offer support and education to families of GLBT patients?

## Coming out to a spouse

◆ *Far From Heaven* (Julianne Moore, Dennis Quaid). This film is set in the 1950s. Cathy (Julianne Moore) is a devoted, seemingly happily married wife and mother of two children. She senses that there is something wrong with her husband, Frank (Dennis Quaid), who seems cold and distant.

a (0:22:30–0:25:15). Cathy pays Frank a surprise visit at work and discovers him in the arms of another man.

1 If Cathy sought your assistance after discovering Frank's homosexuality, what resources would you make available to her?
2 What health risks might exist for Frank and his wife in choosing to conceal his homosexuality?

# Conversion therapy

◆ *Far From Heaven* (Julianne Moore, Dennis Quaid). See previous section on coming out to a spouse for movie description.

a (0:28:35–0:32:55). At Cathy's urging, Frank agrees to undergo psychoanalysis for conversion of his homosexuality.

1 Do you think that homosexuality can be 'changed'?
2 How would you respond to a patient who asked if it was possible to change sexual orientation?

3  How would you handle a GLBT patient who expressed religious conflicts with their sexuality?

b (0:34:12–0:35:28). A close friend's derogatory comment about homosexuals affects Cathy's desire to discuss her concerns and questions about homosexuality.

1  How would you answer Cathy's questions about the prevalence and causes of homosexuality?

c (0:45:45–0:48:30). After excessive drinking, Frank attempts to have sexual relations with Cathy but is unsuccessful. Cathy reassures Frank that it is not his fault. He becomes very angry and slaps Cathy.

1  What impact would the failure of conversion therapy have on Frank and Cathy?
2  What might be the function of Frank's excessive drinking? Would hearing about this incident make you consider referring him for substance abuse treatment? Are there substance abuse resources in your community for gays and lesbians?

## Concealing identity

◆ *Big Eden* (Arye Gross, George Coe, Tim DeKay, Nan Martin). Henry Hart (Arye Gross) is openly gay and living in New York City. He returns to his home town to care for his ailing grandfather, Sam (George Coe). While he is there, he behaves as if he is 'in the closet.'

a (0:23:10–0:26:48). Henry reunites with his best friend and high-school crush, Dean Stewart (Tim DeKay). Dean's conflicts about his sexuality prompted Henry's leaving home and his subsequent therapy. Simultaneously he is dealing with the town's nosy widow, Thayer (Nan Martin), who wants to find him a partner.

1  If Henry was your patient, how would you conduct your medical interview to increase his trust?
2  Would you recommend that Henry disclose to Dean his homosexuality and longstanding crush?

b (1:21:48–1:24:43). His grandfather gives Henry unconditional love and hopes that his grandson will acknowledge his homosexuality.

1  What might be some of the reasons why Henry conceals his sexual identity from his grandfather?

c (1:41:18–1:41:58). Henry regrets not disclosing his sexual orientation to his grandfather before his death.

1  How might Henry resolve his feelings of guilt following his grandfather's death?

## Gender variant behavior

◆ *Torch Song Trilogy* (Matthew Broderick, Harvey Fierstein, Brian Kerwin, Anne Bancroft). Arnold Beckoff (Harvey Fierstein) is a drag queen. He pursues a relationship with Ed (Brian Kerwin), who is bisexual. After the relationship ends, Arnold meets and settles into a very content and committed relationship with Alan (Matthew Broderick). Sadly, their relationship eventually comes to a tragic end. Arnold's mother (Anne Bancroft) struggles to accept her son's homosexuality.

a (0:00:34–0:02:06). Through the use of flashback, we get a glimpse of Arnold as a child. Arnold's mother calls out for her young son. She discovers Arnold in her closet dressed in make-up, jewelery and women's clothing.

1  How would you respond to a mother's concern over her son's preferences for playing with dolls and wearing dresses?
2  How knowledgeable are you with regard to defining various gender-identity terms (e.g. drag queen, transvestite, transsexual)?

# Bisexuality

◆ *Torch Song Trilogy* (Matthew Broderick, Harvey Fierstein, Brian Kerwin, Anne Bancroft). See previous section on gender variant behavior for movie description.

a (0:26:29–0:30:05). Arnold is in a relationship with Ed. He makes a surprise visit to Ed's apartment and discovers that he is dating a woman. Ed reminds Arnold that he is bisexual. Ed's date overhears them talking about their relationship as Arnold is getting on the elevator.

1  What advice would you give to Ed's girlfriend if she came to see you to discuss Ed's homosexual experiences?
2  What knowledge, values and beliefs do you have with regard to bisexuality?

# Suicide

◆ *Torch Song Trilogy* (Matthew Broderick, Harvey Fierstein, Brian Kerwin, Anne Bancroft). See earlier section on gender variant behavior for movie description.

a (0:34:17–0:41:06). Five months after their break-up, Ed shows up in Arnold's dressing room. He misses Arnold and shares a dream with him about his attempted suicide.

1  What would you say to a patient who disclosed that they had had a dream about attempting suicide?

# Hate crimes and victimizations

◆ *Torch Song Trilogy* (Matthew Broderick, Harvey Fierstein, Brian Kerwin, Anne Bancroft). See earlier section on gender variant behavior for movie description.

a (1:11:11–1:18:28). Arnold enjoys a strong and committed relationship with Alan. As Alan is getting take-out food, he hears that an older gay man is being beaten. He rushes to help the man and is attacked himself by a group of unknown men. Arnold sees Alan being taken away by ambulance. Alan dies a victim of hate crime.

1  What types of personal, familial and societal stresses are specific to GLBT patients?
2  How might a GLBT patient manifest stress?

## Moving beyond shame

◆ *Torch Song Trilogy* (Matthew Broderick, Harvey Fierstein, Brian Kerwin, Anne Bancroft). See earlier section on gender variant behavior for movie description.

a  (1:33:25–1:36:50). Arnold and his mother visit his father's grave. Arnold stops at Alan's grave site nearby. Arnold's mother becomes very upset when he prays at his lover's burial site. Arnold becomes very angry towards his mother when she shows little sympathy for his loss.

b  (1:37:23–1:42:54). Arnold and his mother are back at his apartment. He apologizes for losing his temper and wants to talk with her. He wants to adopt a child, but his mother questions his ability to parent a child. In anger, Arnold's mother says that if she had known all the heartache she would endure because of his sexuality, she would not have bothered to have him.

1  How would you approach a mother's shame over having a homosexual son or daughter?
2  How would you respond to a friend who admits to feeling shame about having a homosexual relative?
3  How would you help Arnold's mother understand her son's desire to adopt a child?

c  (1:48:45–1:53:45). Arnold's mother feels that she has been left out of her son's life. She tells him that she wished he had told her about the circumstances surrounding Alan's death. Arnold's mother begins to accept his homosexuality without shame and disapproval.

1  What do you think of what Arnold's mother has said? Is there truth to her argument?

## Aging, grief and losses

◆ *If These Walls Could Talk 2* (Vanessa Redgrave, Marian Seldes, Sharon Stone, Ellen DeGeneres). Edith (Vanessa Redgrave), an aging woman, is left to face prejudice and intolerance after the death of her lifelong lover, Abby (Marian Seldes). There are two other stories in this film, one of which is cited in the following section on same-sex families and children.

a  (0:01:50–0:04:15). Edith and Abby refrain from demonstrating physical affection. A group of teenagers laugh and glare at them.

1  How often do you enquire about the sexual orientation of an older patient?

b  (0:04:22–0:13:30). When Abby is taken to hospital after a fall and dies, Edith experiences additional emotional distress due to having to deny the extent of their relationship. She lacks legal rights to visitation and decision making.

1 What impact would Edith's full disclosure of her relationship with Abby have on her healthcare experience today?

c (0:15:10–0:17:30). Edith 'straightens' their home by removing pictures of her and Abby. Prior to the arrival of Abby's family, Edith moves Abby's clothing and personal belongings to the guest bedroom.

1 What are important considerations for aging gay or lesbian couples?

d (0:20:00–0:28:30). Abby's nephew and his wife come to the home and take away possessions that belong to Edith. Edith suffers alone, confused and distraught, without legal recourse.

1 Are you aware of legal resources to protect the rights of GLBT patients?

## Same-sex families and children

◆ *If These Walls Could Talk 2* (Vanessa Redgrave, Marian Seldes, Sharon Stone, Ellen DeGeneres). See previous section on aging, grief and losses for movie description.

a (1:29:35–1:31:50). Fran (Sharon Stone) and Kal (Ellen DeGeneres) use artificial insemination to become pregnant. They discuss the possible stigma that their unborn child may face due to having lesbian parents.

1 How would you respond to Fran's concerns and questions about their child having lesbian parents?
2 What does research conclude about the psychological adjustment of children raised by gay and lesbian parents?
3 Where would you refer same-sex parents for information on raising children?

## HIV/AIDS

◆ *Philadelphia* (Tom Hanks, Denzel Washington). Andrew Beckett (Tom Hanks) has a promising career as an attorney with a major law firm until his partners discover that he has AIDS. He seeks legal representation from Joe Miller (Denzel Washington) after the firm dismisses him for 'incompetence.'

a (0:21:38–0:28:55). Despite Joe Miller's 'ambulance-chaser' practice, he recoils physically from shaking Andrew's hand, and he rejects the case immediately after learning of Andrew's illness and homosexual orientation.

b (0:29:38–0:32:38). After Andrew's visit, Joe rushes to his family physician with concerns about HIV contamination. At home with his wife and newborn daughter, Joe is righteous about his bigotry, homophobia and 'caricatures' of the homosexual community. His wife counters his stereotypic views with the names of close gay friends – construction workers, and her aunt, who Joe states is too sensual and voluptuous to be a lesbian.

c (0:33:00–0:40:55). In a legal library, Joe Miller witnesses discrimination against Andrew, which makes him reconsider and accept Andrew's case.

1  How would you support a patient after diagnosing HIV/AIDS?
2  How could you prepare a patient for possible public and familial judgement, rejection and discrimination?
3  What resources exist in your community to assist with legal and psychological issues?

## Transgender

◆ *Boys Don't Cry* (Hilary Swank, Peter Sargaard, Brendan Sexton III, Chloe Sevigny). This is the true story of Teena Brandon (Hilary Swank), a woman who feels that, despite her biology, she is emotionally a man (transgender), and is known as Brandon when presenting as a male.

a  (0:01:30–0:06:30). Brandon prepares for his first meeting with a girl. Boys later chase him after discovering that he is biologically female.

b  (0:17:10–0:22:10). Brandon is able to trust and bond with John (Peter Sarsgaard) and Tom (Brendan Sexton III).

c  (0:31:05–0:32:20). Brandon hides his biological sex.

d  (0:51:08–0:52:30). Brandon shares his wish to marry Lana (Chloe Sevigny) with a close friend, who tries to dissuade him.

e  (0:53:13–1:00:21). Brandon makes love to Lana, who grows suspicious of Brandon's biological sex.

f  (1:24:00–1:34:40). A police interview and medical examination are conducted after John and Tom rape and beat Brandon.

g  (1:28:12–1:42:25). Lana loves and accepts Brandon for who he is.

h  (1:47:35–1:50:25). Brandon is murdered.

1  What challenges exist in the 'coming out' process for transgendered individuals? How might it compare to and differ from the process for gay and lesbian individuals?
2  How well are you able to understand the emotional issues faced by transsexuals?
3  What resources are available to help transsexuals with their personal and workplace transitions?

## Reference

1.  Harrison AE. Primary care of lesbian and gay patients: educating ourselves and our students. *Fam Med* 1996; **28**: 10–23.

# Chapter 24

# Complementary and alternative medicine

*Wadie Najm and Patricia Lenahan*

Complementary and alternative medicine (CAM) incorporate healthcare approaches that are not part of the dominant medical system. Between 30 and 60% of the US population currently use CAM for disease prevention and/or management of disease conditions.[1] Popular interest in CAM has sparked research in this area and improved the availability of products and resources. However, many healthcare providers' perspective on CAM, including its use and potential abuse, is limited by inadequate education and exposure. In today's world an essential component of providing comprehensive medical care increasingly includes heightened awareness and knowledge of and ability to communicate about CAM. In this chapter the authors present clips from several movies that address a number of different aspects of CAM. These scenes can be used as triggers for more comprehensive discussions about CAM.

## Home remedies

◆ *Doc Hollywood* (Michael J Fox, Julie Warner, Woody Harrelson). This is a movie about a young physician, Ben Stone (Michael J Fox), whose trip to plastic surgery residency training in Beverly Hills takes a detour through the small town of Grady, South Carolina, where he is pressured to provide general medical care at the community clinic.

a (0:24:20–0:25:20). In this scene Dr Stone is caring for a patient who used a home remedy to treat a cut on his toe.

1 How would you approach this patient?
2 How do you discuss the use of home remedies or CAM with your patients?
3 Discuss the different types of CAM.

## Diets and dietary supplements

◆ *Safe* (Julianne Moore). Carol (Julianne Moore) is a suburban housewife who begins to develop vague physical complaints that are initially thought to be the result of fatigue and stress. She undergoes a series of allergy tests and is referred to a psychiatrist to help her to deal with her stress. After Carol suffers a seizure due to the chemicals at her dry cleaners, she is admitted to a medical hospital and eventually to a specialized treatment facility for chemically sensitive patients.

a (0:55:50–1:02:00). Carol attends a meeting with a group that discusses the chemically sensitive person. Later, at lunch with a friend, she talks about how things such as 'make-up' now affect her. The scene then shifts to Carol listening to a tape recommending fasting and adjustment of one's living conditions to eliminate mold and certain foods as a safe way to clear one's body of impurities. The tape recommends that the fast be followed by the rotation diet or the rare foods diet.

1  What do you know about the rotary diversified diet (RDD)? Would you recommend this as a treatment for a patient who is experiencing multiple sensitivities to food?
2  What foods are considered to be 'bad' foods? How does this compare with the situation for patients from other cultures who consider foods (and medicines) to be either 'hot' or 'cold'? What implications do such beliefs have for treatment?
3  How would you counsel a patient who approaches you about the benefits of popular diets (e.g. Atkins diet, South Beach diet, Hawaiian diet, Zone diet)?
4  What advice can you give a patient who will only eat organic foods?
5  What is the role of emotional support in recovery from illness?

◆ *Lorenzo's Oil* (Nick Nolte, Susan Sarandon). This is a movie based on the true story of Augusto Odone (Nick Nolte) and his wife, Michaela (Susan Sarandon), who fight to save the life of their son Lorenzo. Lorenzo is diagnosed in early 1984 with adrenoleukodystrophy (ALD), an inborn error of metabolism. After several failed therapies, the parents realize that Lorenzo's care is beyond the help of conventional medicine, and they begin their own investigation of the disease and a quest for a cure.

a (1:00:59–1:03:00). In this scene, seven months after Lorenzo has been diagnosed with ALD, his parents find a purified form of olive oil that their research has convinced them would help to treat Lorenzo. The mother is contacting a company in order to obtain this oil.

1  Discuss the difference between what scientists and the public would accept as evidence-based medicine.
2  Discuss the regulations overseeing dietary supplements and what consumers can do to ensure a safe product.

## Health beliefs

◆ *Soul Food* (Vanessa Williams, Vivica A Fox, Nia Long, Brandon Hammond, Irma P Hall). The story of an extended family who share Sunday dinner, family values, traditions and secrets.

a (0:12:16–0:12:52). Big Mama (Irma P Hall) is at the stove and does not realize that she has burned her arm. Her daughter says that she bets Big Mama is not taking her insulin, and she asks when she last saw her doctor. Big Mama replies that she does not need a doctor, just her salve, turpentine and herbs.

1  What health beliefs are demonstrated in this scene?
2  How would you integrate Big Mama's belief system into your treatment plan?
3  How can you best take a history of CAM beliefs and practices from your patients?

# Spirituality

◆ *Lorenzo's Oil* (Nick Nolte, Susan Sorandon). See earlier section on diets and dietary supplements for movie description.

a (0:05:44–0:13:45). In this scene Lorenzo starts to experience the initial symptoms of ALD. The medical community struggles with his diagnosis. The family is confused and agrees to admit Lorenzo to hospital for additional testing.

1 Discuss the role of faith and prayer in healing and healthcare.
2 If you were the parent of a child with ALD, how likely might you be to seek out and utilize CAM?

# Mind–body dilemmas in healthcare

◆ *Safe* (Julianne Moore). See earlier section on diets and dietary supplements for movie description.

a (1:06:40–1:11:60). Carol decides to enter the Wrenwood Center, a facility that specifically treats environmental illnesses. She wears a mask around her neck and is using oxygen. Upon her arrival, a staff member takes her on a tour of the facility and tells her that it is a chemical-free zone.

1 As a healthcare professional, what are your reactions to the Wrenwood Center?
2 Carol displays many of the symptoms associated with multiple chemical sensitivities (MCS) and idiopathic environmental intolerance (IEI) (e.g. hoarseness, fatigue, cough, cognitive change and mood dysfunction). How would you diagnose and treat these symptoms?
3 Carol was referred to a psychiatrist prior to her admission to Wrenwood Center. What alternative treatment modalities might have been employed to alleviate Carol's symptoms?
4 How do you think Carol feels about her decision to enter the Wrenwood Center? What level of distress and disability does Carol experience?
5 How would you discuss issues such as pediatric immunizations with a mother who, like Carol, is fearful of environmental toxins?

b (0:37:32–1:43:08). Peter, the founder of the Wrenwood Center, is conducting a group counseling session. He suggests that anger and other unpleasant emotions are frequent contributors to a person's immune system becoming damaged. He encourages the patients to remember their affirmations.

1 What are the effects of stress and anger on the immune system?
2 How would you counsel a patient with an environmental illness about lifestyle changes? What changes would you recommend?
3 What psychiatric conditions or diagnoses might you consider, as part of your differential diagnosis, for a patient who complains of MCS or IEI?
4 What aspects of integrative medicine (e.g. yoga, meditation, tai chi) might be beneficial to Carol?

## Reference

1. Wootton JC, Sparber A. Surveys of complementary and alternative medicine usage: a review of general population trends and specific patient populations. *Semin Integr Med* 2003; 1: 10–24.

Chapter 25

# Cultural diversity

*Kathleen A Culhane-Pera and Jeffrey Ring*

The road to becoming a culturally responsive physician is paved with the personal and professional development of *awareness* (of personal vulnerability to bias and stereotyping), *knowledge* (of other cultural ways, world views and health beliefs) and *skills* (of doctor–patient communication and negotiation of treatment strategies). The inclusion of film clips in this area of teaching can be helpful, particularly in increasing cultural awareness and knowledge. However, family practice educators must be very careful to instruct learners on the perils of making fixed generalizations about their patients and other people based solely on video segments. Cultural video viewing must be framed as material for the generation of hypotheses about patients from different backgrounds, and *not* as definitive portrayals of universal group characteristics or experiences. As such, the debriefing discussions of these video clips assume primary importance and must address both the richness and the limitations of the film portrayals in applications to the clinical setting.

We have organized the listings in this chapter by categories of ethnic and cultural group, recognizing that people's cultural identity is a complex matter which makes these terms rather problematic. The film scenes in each section deal with some aspects of culture that could be considered for people in all groups, such as ethnic identity, stereotypes, discrimination, acculturation, gender, family expectations, healing, religious beliefs, and conflicts with people from other ethnic and cultural groups. All of these issues are pertinent to the care of patients from diverse backgrounds in clinical settings.[1-4]

## Cultural diversity

### African American

◆ *Soul Food* (Vanessa Williams, Vivica A Fox, Nia Long, Brandon Hammond, Irma P Hall). This is a film about the Joseph family narrated by a grandson, Ahmad (Brandon Hammond).

a (0:02:35–0:08:06). In these initial scenes the family celebrates the youngest sister's wedding (at which 'skeletons in the closet' appear), and then gathers for Sunday dinner at the house of Big Mama (Irma P Hall).

1 What are the directors of this film portraying about the way people celebrate? In what way does this scene remind you of the way that your family celebrates? What is similar and what is different?

2 What does Big Mama do that illustrates how she 'cares for everyone in the family'?

3 Why is the film entitled *Soul Food*? What does the phrase 'soul food' mean to you? What foods are important for your family? What social, emotional and historical significance does food have in ethnicity and family?

4 Did you understand the family's speech? What is Ebonics? What is its language origin and structure? Do you consider this to be a 'legitimate' language? Do you think it should be taught in schools? Do you speak in Ebonics to people who speak it to you in the clinical setting? Why or why not? In what way is speaking Ebonics similar to speaking Spanglish to people who speak it to you in the clinical setting?

## Additional scenes

a (0:08:16–0:10:04, 0:12:00–0:15:03, 0:16:55–0:19:55). This scene shows Sunday dinner, with a description of food and its meaning.

## Asian American

◆ *Snow Falling on Cedars* (Ethan Hawke, Youki Kudoh). This is a film about the murder trial of a Japanese-American defendant in the Pacific Northwest just after the Japanese relocation and internment events of World War Two. It also portrays the ethnic identity challenges of a Japanese-American teenager amidst social prejudices and mores about multicultural relationships.

a (0:27:50–0:29:05). This scene depicts a discussion between a teenage girl, Hatsue Imada (Youki Kudoh), and her mother about dating Japanese or European-American boys.

b (0:54:40–0:55:48). This scene shows Hatsue reacting strongly to her mother's admonishments, and yelling 'I don't want to be Japanese!'.

1 What differences do you observe between Hatsue and her mother with regard to their own ethnic identities and attitudes towards Anglo-American people?

2 Why is Hatsue's mother so adamant about Hatsue not dating Ishmael Chambers?

3 What are the emotional and physical consequences of racism and prejudice for minorities in this country?

## European American

◆ *Keeping the Faith* (Ben Stiller, Edward Norton, Jenna Elfman, Anne Bancroft). This is a romantic comedy that portrays the parallel professional and personal development of two childhood friends who become a priest and a rabbi, respectively, and the changes over time in their relationships with a female childhood friend.

a (0:10:24–0:13:23). This scene shows a series of increasingly successful attempts by both young men to grow into their spiritual leader roles.

1 What are the similarities and differences between these two men in terms of their approaches to their work and to their roles as spiritual leaders?

2   What is meant by the term 'white privilege'? Do you see any reflections of this concept in the film clip?
3   What are the potential implications of Jewish and Catholic beliefs for healthcare and the doctor–patient relationship?

## Latino American

◆ *My Family – Mi Familia* (Jimmy Smits, Esai Morales, Eduardo Lopez Rojas, Jenny Gago, Elpidia Carrillo, Lupe Ontiveros). This film by Mexican Americans traces three generations of the Sanchez family from the 1920s through the turbulent 1950s to the stark realities of the present day.

a (0:11:40–0:23:40). During a purge of 'illegal' workers, a pregnant woman is deported from California to Mexico, despite the fact that she is a citizen. On the journey back to her family, she and her infant son cross a river and almost drown. The infant is subsequently given a curing ceremony for *susto* (fright).

1   Why were the 'Mexicans' being deported? What is the history of North-western Mexico becoming the Southwestern USA? What is the historical relationship between the two countries with regard to migration and migrant workers?
2   What is *susto*? What is the traditional treatment for *susto*? How is *susto* being manifested, considered and treated in the USA now?
3   What is the range of emotions experienced during immigration? How have people migrated to the USA? How have they been received? In what ways is the USA a melting pot? What other images/metaphors describe the cultural diversity of the USA?
4   What are the effects on health and mental health of anti-immigrant attitudes and racism in society?

## Additional scene

a (1:46:24–1:50:52). A law-student son introduces his Anglo fiancée and her parents to his family.

## Native American

◆ *Smoke Signals* (Adam Beach, Evan Adams, Gary Farmer). This is a movie about Thomas (Evan Adams) and Victor (Adam Beach), two young Native American men from the Coeur D'Alene reservation who share a journey from Idaho to Arizona after the death of Victor's father, Arnold Joseph (Gary Farmer).

a (0:15:15–0:20:20). This scene shows the beginning of a spiritual journey as Victor comes to Thomas's house and tells him that he can join the trip (with certain conditions) as they walk along a road and hitch a ride from two young women.

1   What are the directors saying about the ethnic identity of young Native Americans on this reservation?

2   What stereotypes are they depicting? What range of characteristics are they portraying?

3   What do you learn about your stereotypes of this group? Do these images dispel or reinforce your stereotypes?

4   In what way is America a foreign country, 'as foreign as it gets'?

5   What do you know about the history of Native American people, the creation and existence of reservations, and the health of Native Americans on and off the reservations?

### Additional scenes

a   (0:34:30–0:37:56). In this scene on a bus, there is a discussion concerning what is a 'real' Indian.

b   (1:09:40–1:12:18). In this scene with a policeman it is questioned whether people can be real Indians if they do not drink alcohol.

## Cultural diversity and end-of-life issues

*See* Chapter 8 for additional films in this subject area.

◆ *The Road Home* (Zhang Ziyi, Sun Honglei). This is a movie about a wife's desire to have a traditional funeral procession for her dead husband, despite logistical barriers and community opposition.

a   (0:01:45–0:10:00). In this scene, a grown-up son arrives home after his father's death and discovers his mother's wishes regarding his father's funeral and burial.

1   What importance does this widow attach to the traditional burial procedures? Why do you think this is important to her but not to others?

2   What funeral and burial practices are important to you, to people with your religious perspective and to people from your traditional ethnic background? What changes have occurred over time?

3   What interactions have you had with families from various ethnic backgrounds at the time of death and dying?

### Additional scene

a   (1:11:30–1:14:30). This scene shows the funeral procession and grave.

### Additional film

◆ *Ju Dou* (Li Gong, Baotian Li, Wei Li, Zhang Yi, Jia Zhaoji) includes a remarkable scene of a funeral procession in a Chinese feudal society, in which mourners are actively and physically involved in attempting to block a death procession carrying the casket and deceased to the grave site.

# Cultural diversity and gay, lesbian, bisexual and transgendered issues

*See* Chapter 23 for additional films in this content area.

## Chinese gay American

◆ *The Wedding Banquet* (Winston Chao, May Chin, Mitchell Lichtenstein). This is a film about a gay couple, Gao (Winston Chao), a Chinese man, and Simon (Mitchell Lichtenstein), a European American.

a (0:00:00–0:12:07). The opening scenes reveal Gao's parents' expectations that he will marry a Chinese woman, and his struggle about whether or not to tell his parents that he is gay.

1 What struggles does Gao have with regard to 'coming out' to his parents? Why do you think this seems to be more difficult for him than for Simon?
2 What issues arise for gay/lesbian/bisexual individuals when 'coming out' to families, friends and society in general? In what ways are 'coming-out' issues similar and different in various ethnic and religious groups? Can you identify potential unique social stressors for gay and lesbian individuals who are also from ethnic minorities?
3 How do Gao's parents see Wei Wei (May Chin), Wai Tung's presumed fiancée? What gender roles and stereotypes are portrayed? How accurate or inaccurate are these stereotypes as generalities?
4 This film clip also depicts struggles for illegal immigrants migrating from China to the USA. What do you know about the smuggling of people from Asia and other countries to the USA? How does immigrant status influence their health and their ability to receive healthcare?

## Additional scenes

a (0:23:40–0:25:16). Gao's parents arrive and meet Gao, Simon and Wei Wei.

b (0:49:49–0:52:49). This clip shows wedding scenes between Gao and Wei Wei.

c (1:20:11–1:24:50). Gao tells his mother that he is gay while his father is in hospital.

## References

1. National Video Resources. *Viewing Race: a videography and resource guide;* www. viewingrace.org. Videoform publication. Accessed 18 February 2003.
2. Summerfield E, Lee S. *Seeing the Big Picture: exploring American cultures on film.* Yarmouth, MA: Intercultural Press Inc, 2001.
3. Summerfield E. *Crossing Cultures Through Film.* Yarmouth, MA: Intercultural Press Inc, 1993.
4. Zeigler L. *Film and Video Resources for International Educational Exchange.* Yarmouth, MA: Intercultural Press Inc, 2000.

Chapter 26

# Physical and mental disabilities

*Layne Prest, Kathleen A Culhane-Pera, Jeffrey Ring and Patricia Lenahan*

The Americans with Disabilities Act (1990) defines disability as a physical or mental impairment that substantially limits one or more major life activities. Individuals with developmental disabilities are born with or acquire a disability before the age of 18 years. Cerebral palsy, spina bifida, mental retardation and autism are all examples of developmental disabilities.

The importance of screening, early detection and intervention for developmental disabilities cannot be over-emphasized. Early intervention can dramatically alter an affected child's course and health outcome. Parents depend upon primary healthcare providers to recognize problems in childhood development and to identify risk factors that place children at risk for such disabilities. It is paramount for providers to be aware of resources in the community which can assist families in the evaluation, treatment and support of children with disabilities. Such resources include schools, county regional centers, physical and occupational therapy, and specialty treatment centers.

Physical disabilities acquired in adulthood may result from medical, neurological and/or traumatic conditions. They can dramatically alter bodily integrity, self-esteem and function, and require extensive occupational and social adaptation. Again, physicians and other specialists can make significant contributions to the treatment and adjustment of individuals facing such challenges.

This chapter presents film clips about several types of disability, both physical and mental.

## Autism

◆ *Down in the Delta* (Alfre Woodard, Al Freeman Jr, Mary Alice, Esther Rolle, Wesley Snipes, Loretta Devine). This film was directed by Maya Angelou and depicts the struggles of a young African-American woman, Loretta (Alfre Woodard), who is living in Chicago with her mother, Rosa (Mary Alice), and her two children, one of whom is autistic. On her mother's insistence, Loretta agrees to spend the summer 'down in the delta' with her two children, visiting her Uncle Earl (Al Freeman Jr) and her Aunt Annie (Esther Rolle), who has Alzheimer's disease. Loretta learns much about herself and her family in the process.

a (0:27:04–0:28:22). Loretta and the children are on the bus. You can hear Tracy, Loretta's autistic daughter, screaming in the background. Two women exiting the bus exhibit their displeasure. Loretta is met at the bus stop by her Uncle Earl (Al Freeman Jr), who asks why a big girl like Tracy needs to sleep in a crib. Uncle Earl looks at Tracy, who lashes out at both of them. Loretta tells him that Tracy goes crazy if anyone looks her in the eye.

b (0:52:32–0:54:07). Loretta is visiting Zenia (Loretta Devine), her aunt's caretaker. She asks Zenia what she sees when she looks at Tracy. Zenia replies that she could be a crack baby. Loretta explains that Tracy is autistic. Zenia then turns the tables on Loretta and asks her what she thinks Tracy sees when she looks at Loretta. Zenia says she sees her mother.

c (1:14:02–1:14:40). Uncle Earl and Loretta are saying goodbye to Annie. As she walks past Tracy's crib, Tracy waves and says 'bye-bye' to her mother. Loretta lifts her up and hugs her tightly. Tracy says 'bye-bye' when her mother leaves.

1   What are some public misperceptions about autism? (In this film, there was an assumption that the child was a 'crack baby'.)
2   What is the current thinking regarding the cause(s) of autism? How would you explain the cause of autism to a parent?
3   How would you respond to a parent(s) who refused vaccines for their child because of concern that vaccines are associated with the development of autism?
4   What community resources are available for children with autism and their families?

## Neurological disorders

### Amyotrophic lateral sclerosis (ALS)

◆ *The Theory of Flight* (Helena Bonham Carter, Kenneth Branagh). Jane (Helena Bonham Carter) is a young woman who has been diagnosed with ALS and is now confined to a wheelchair. Social services have been trying to find volunteers to provide respite for her mother, who is her primary caregiver. Richard (Kenneth Branagh) is sentenced by the court to perform community service, and is assigned to provide companionship for Jane.

a (0:04:36–0:08:20). Richard is met by the social worker, who introduces him to Jane. She explains that Jane's voice has begun to deteriorate and that she is being encouraged to use her speech machine more. The social worker adds that Jane is 'all there' mentally. After their introduction, Richard asks Jane what she usually likes to do. Jane merely rolls her eyes. Richard and Jane go outside, where Jane shares her observations about people who volunteer (all of them are desperately lonely) and the feelings that people have while walking next to her wheelchair.

1   What feelings does Jane evoke in the people around her?
2   How difficult is it to understand Jane's speech? How could this affect doctor–patient communication?
3   What are some common reactions to seeing people in wheelchairs?
4   How is the power dynamic in relationships and communication affected by one's being in a wheelchair?

b (0:13:03–0:15:46). Richard has taken Jane on an outing to a museum, where she appears bored. He asks her what she wants to do, and she suggests going on a carnival ride. Richard immediately says that it is impossible, but then relents.

Initially Jane is laughing and appears quite happy, but then she begins to cry. The scene ends with Jane going to the emergency room where she is treated and then discharged.

1 What are the issues for disabled people participating in activities such as these?
2 What are the reactions of able-bodied individuals with regard to the inclusion of disabled people in these activities?
3 Was Jane's ultimate reaction and need for medical treatment a predictable outcome? Did it tend to confirm Richard's view that Jane should not engage in these activities?

## Cerebral palsy

◆ *My Left Foot* (Daniel Day-Lewis, Brenda Fricker, Hugh O'Conor). This is a dramatization of Christy Brown's autobiography, which chronicles his life as a man with spastic cerebral palsy.

a (0:10:15–0:15:38). In this series of scenes, Christy (Hugh O'Conor and later Daniel Day-Lewis) is a seven-year-old boy who is being fed by his mother. He tries to help his mother after she falls down the stairs, and is then alternately pitied and ridiculed by neighbors who come to her rescue.

1 What are your initial reactions to Christy Brown? What impressions do you have of his character and of his potential, particularly with regard to his intellectual and artistic capabilities?
2 How do his mother and neighbors feel towards Christy, and how do they assess his abilities? In general, how do family and community members assess people with handicaps?

b (0:29:55–0:31:23). Christy is seen playing soccer with his brothers and boys from the neighborhood.

c (0:47:20–0:47:40). Christy is expressing his anger towards his father through his painting.

d (1:03:40–1:07:13). Christy's paintings are being shown in a gallery.

e (1:07:13–1:12:15). Christy discovers that his desired girlfriend is engaged.

1 After viewing these scenes, how do your impressions of Christy's abilities change over time?
2 Do you think that he deserves success as a painter and writer?
3 Do you think that he deserves and/or can find happiness in a romantic relationship?
4 In general, how do our impressions of others blind us to their true potential?
5 How do you think Christy's environment (social, physical and cultural) influenced his personal development?

# Tic disorders

## Tourette's disorder

◆ *Niagara, Niagara* (Robin Tunney, Henry Thomas, Michael Parks). This is a story of two 'misfit' teenagers who find each other and search for meaning in their lives. Seth (Henry Thomas) is the son of an abusive father who meets Marcie (Robin Tunney) in a drugstore. Both are shoplifting. Marcie suffers from Tourette's disorder, which she tries to control with alcohol in addition to her medications.

a (0:04:20–0:06:12). Marcie and Seth are getting into Seth's car after leaving the drugstore and Marcie suddenly jerks back, falling on the ground and engaging in some behavioral rituals. As she gets out of the car she swears at Seth and then repeats the word 'sorry' numerous times.

1 What is the impact of Tourette's disorder on adolescent development?
2 How is Tourette's disorder classified according to the DSM-IV TR?
3 What is the impact of Tourette's disorder on self-esteem?
4 How is Tourette's disorder viewed by the general public?

b (0:18:48–0:22:30). Marcie talks to Seth about her diagnosis and the impact that it had on her at school. She talks very clinically about symptoms such as echolalia, which she explains to Seth. Marcie says that she does not want to be like this. She tells Seth that both alcohol and sex help to relieve the symptoms along with her medications (Haldol and Cogentin). Marcie says that she was trying to 'hold in' her tics because she did not want to scare Seth. She adds that she tries to incorporate her tics into what she does.

1 How has Marcie attempted to cope with her illness?
2 How would you interpret her very clinical explanation of her illness?

c (0:25:50–0:29:12). Marcie is trying to obtain her medications, and hands the pharmacist a prescription for Motrin. Marcie is seen rewriting the prescription at a bar.

1 Have you ever had patients who attempted to rewrite prescriptions?
2 Marcie takes both Haldol and Cogentin. How frequently are these drugs abused?
3 What is the pharmacist's response? How does he view Marcie's attempts to rewrite a prescription?

d (0:31:44–0:38:10). This scene shows Marcie and Seth stopping at various pharmacies in an attempt to get her prescription refilled. One pharmacist confronts the teenagers and says that he is an expert at identifying drug-addicted kids. The stress of this encounter results in Marcie having an attack. Later, Marcie and Seth are seen breaking into the pharmacy.

1 How do you identify drug-addicted children/adolescents?
2 What is the impact of stress on Tourette's disorder?

# Deafness

◆ *Sound and Fury* (Nita Artinian, Peter Artinian). This is a documentary that focuses on an extended family with three generations of both hearing and deaf family members. Family members are shown deciding whether or not to obtain cochlear implants for two children.

a (0:25:18–0:33:15, 0:42:10–0:44:03). In this series of scenes, deaf parents and their deaf daughter meet hearing parents and a deaf child with a cochlear implant. The deaf mother argues with her hearing sister-in-law, and the deaf mother and her deaf daughter talk about deaf culture.

1 What do the hearing parents say is important about hearing? Why did they decide in favor of the cochlear implant?
2 What do the deaf parents say is important about being deaf? Why did they decide against the implant?
3 What is deaf culture? What do 'self-esteem' and 'identity' as a deaf child mean? What are the important ingredients of 'culture'? What happens when people lose essential ingredients of culture?

# Paralysis

◆ *Passion Fish* (Mary McDonnell, Alfre Woodard). Mary McDonnell portrays Mary-Alice Culhane, a television star who is permanently disabled while in the prime of her career. After being struck by a passing car, she is left a paraplegic. This movie depicts Mary-Alice's reaction to this crisis in her life, including her initial adjustment and eventual adaptation. This process involves not only coping with physical incapacity, but also having to adjust to the loss of fame, status and general role functioning as a woman. After the immediate crisis and some rehabilitation, Mary-Alice returns to her family home in Louisiana (a place to which she had vowed she would never return) and becomes a recluse. A series of caregivers come and go before she is joined by Chantelle (Alfre Woodard), an African-American woman from the inner city who is in the midst of working through her own life crises (drug addiction, loss of custody of her child and estrangement from her family). Together the two women create a relatively healthy interdependent relationship, which becomes the crucible for their individual healing.

a (0:00:00–0:06:21). This scene shows the initial crisis and Mary-Alice's reactions.

1 What signs of grief are evident in the 'patient'?
2 What losses has Mary-Alice experienced?
3 How is Mary-Alice's difficulty in adjusting being manifested in her life?
4 What psychological defenses and coping mechanisms does Mary-Alice use?

b (0:18:06–0:23:01). In this scene Chantelle, the new caregiver, arrives.

1 How are the dynamics between Mary-Alice and Chantelle different from those of previous relationships?
2 How does Chantelle help Mary-Alice to confront the reality of her situation?

3 What is the difference between adjustment and adaptation in response to a permanent disability?

4 How can patients and family members avoid having their lives overtaken or 'saturated' by the impact of disability?

## Mental retardation[1]

◆ *Molly* (Elisabeth Shue, Jill Hennessey, DW Moffett, Aaron Eckhart, Thomas Jane). This is the story of Molly (Elisabeth Shue), a 28-year-old woman who has been living in a nursing home since her parents' death. The facility where she lives is closing down, and her brother Buck (Aaron Eckhart) must now assume responsibility for her care.

a (0:03:10–0:05:25). Buck arrives at the nursing home and meets with the physician, who tells him that they are unsure of Molly's diagnosis. She is either mentally retarded or autistic. The physician says that Molly displays minor savant-like characteristics.

1 How well does the physician's description of Molly's condition help her brother to understand her care needs?

2 How would you provide information to a family member who is unfamiliar with a relative's condition?

b (0:06:20–0:07:00). Buck brings Molly home. She becomes incontinent, and Buck says that this was not part of the deal. He does not know what to do to assist Molly, or how to cope with the incontinence.

1 What is the effect of incontinence on family caregivers?

2 What advice would you give Buck, a young man, on coping with his sister's incontinence?

c (0:16:14–0:17:10). Buck has lost his job because of Molly.

1 What options would be available to care for someone like Molly in the community?

2 What services or resources would you recommend to Buck?

d (0:26:34–0:27:39). Buck and Molly are leaving the Kerran Institute and Buck's car will not start. He becomes frustrated and, as Molly complains repeatedly of feeling cold, Buck yells at her and tells her to shut up. Several nurses and aides are standing outside and observe the interchange. Buck apologizes to Molly.

1 What are the risk factors for abuse?

2 What advice or guidance would you offer a caregiver in a similar situation?

3 What services would be helpful in reducing caregiver stress?

## Self-injury

◆ *28 Days* (Sandra Bullock, Reni Santoni). Gwen (Sandra Bullock) ruins her sister's wedding after arriving drunk. She ends up in a 28-day inpatient program for alcoholics and addicts.

a (0:10:28–0:11:58). A group of patients are sitting at lunch when Daniel (Reni Santoni) angrily asks what the new patient is looking at. He challenges her and says 'Haven't you ever seen a trach scar?'. He then leaves the table. The other patients explain that Daniel did this to himself. He was a physician who used to make himself vomit so that he would not be hung over in the morning. After a recent binge, he began to aspirate and had to perform the tracheotomy himself.

1   What are the effects of visible scars on a patient's self-image?
2   What are the effects of visible scars on other people's perceptions of the patient?
3   How does the fact that Daniel's scar results from drinking affect his emotional state?
4   How would you respond to Daniel's angry outburst?

## Reference

1.   Daily DK, Ardinger HH, Holmes GE. Identification and evaluation of mental retardation. *Am Fam Physician* 2000; **61**: 1059–67.

# Part VI

## Research

# Chapter 27

# A graduate survey of cinemeducation

*Matthew Alexander*

In an effort to provide further evidence with regard to the usefulness of a film-based curriculum, this author recently conducted a survey of graduates from the south eastern family practice residency program with which he is affiliated. The survey assessed graduates' perceptions of the value of using film as a teaching tool.

## Methods

### Sample and survey procedure

Questionnaires (*see* Appendix 2) were sent to all 64 graduates dating back ten years to the time when movie clips were first introduced into the behavioral medicine teaching program. The questionnaire itself was developed in consultation with the research director for the program. Respondents were guaranteed confidentiality. Second and third mailings were sent to non-respondents.

### Survey instrument

Respondents were asked to provide their gender, age and year of graduation. They were then asked to respond to six questions, the first three of which asked for feedback about their behavioral medicine curriculum in general, and the last three of which asked for feedback about the use of film clips during that curriculum in particular. This study focused on responses to the latter three film-related questions.

Respondents were given a trigger statement related to the curriculum, and were then asked to quantify their assessment by circling a number on a Likert scale ranging from 1 (strong disagreement) to 10 (strong agreement). Respondents were also asked to provide written feedback to open-ended questions following each item.

## Data analysis

Ranges and mean scores were developed for each of the three Likert-scale questions studied. Emergent themes were identified by content analysis of the responses to the open-ended questions. These themes were then defined and categorized.

# Results

## Respondents

After three mailings, 39 responses were received, corresponding to a response rate of 61%. However, eight questionnaires were disqualified because respondents were unable to recall films being used in their curriculum. Seven out of eight of *these* respondents belonged to earlier-graduating classes, which had considerably less exposure to popular cinema in their behavioral medicine curriculum than later classes.

## Trigger questions

The three trigger statements and associated open-ended questions that address film curricula are listed below. The number of responses to each question, the mean, the response range and the percentage responding at or over a cut-off value of 8 are included after each trigger statement.

1 The use of film clips increased my enjoyment of the behavioral medicine curriculum. ($n = 30$, mean = 8.8, range = 5–10, responding at cut-off of 8 or higher = 83%). In what ways?
2 The use of film clips improved my retention of behavioral medicine concepts. ($n = 30$, mean = 7.5, range = 3–10, responding at cut-off of 8 or higher = 60%). In what areas?
3 I would recommend expansion of the use of film clips in behavioral medicine seminars ($n = 28$, mean = 7.8, range = 2–10, responding at cut-off of 8 or higher = 64%). Why or why not?

## Open-ended questions

Qualitative analysis yielded the following themes.

1 *Film clips are fun.* Graduates perceived the film clips as an enjoyable and welcome break from traditional didactic approaches. The open-ended questions generated comments such as 'Spiced up routine,' 'Movies are fun and educational' and 'Makes good and fun examples of common problems in life.' Respondents also made comments such as 'I personally have a hard time focusing for 15–20 minutes on lectures, reading, etc., and this is a fresh way to break up the monotony and perhaps enhance the learning experience' and remarked that a film clip 'adds variety to the curriculum.'
2 *Film clips are remembered.* Graduates perceived film clips and the material associated with them as being easy to retain. Comments noted from the survey included 'Visual is remembered better,' 'Popular culture tends to be easily remembered and it stimulates parts of the brain most medical topics cannot,' 'It emphasized the point in memorable ways with living, demonstrated examples' and 'A picture says a thousand words and stays in one's memory longer.'
3 *Film clips are only* part *of an overall behavioral medicine curriculum.* Graduates perceived the need to balance film clips with other methods of behavioral

medicine learning. Sample comments in this context included 'You learn more by doing than by watching,' 'I often felt like it was not an accurate assessment of a typical patient encounter' and 'Film clips can be useful, but you need to be careful that the film clips don't over-simplify things (diagnosis and treatments).'

# Discussion

Taken together, the quantitative and qualitative data support the hypothesis that film clips were viewed by graduates as useful, enjoyable and impactful aspects of their behavioral medicine education. Respondents expressed significant enthusiasm about the use of cinema as an important *part* of their behavioral medicine teaching program, as well as a preference for the current level of its use being either maintained or expanded.

## Study limitations and recommendations

The response rate to the questionnaire was slightly higher than 60%. This is favorable when compared with general expectations in the literature of between 60% and 70% for a response rate to three mailings. Like other similar types of survey study, this analysis relied on self-report data. Such data are prone to several forms of response bias. In an effort to reduce the possible tendency of respondents to skew their responses positively in order to please the investigator (who was also their instructor), the covering letter for the questionnaire guaranteed anonymity and clearly stated that the purpose of the study was to improve the curriculum in the residency. However, in the future a network of residencies could work together to evaluate each other's learners in order to reduce or eliminate such types of bias.

# Part VII

## Additional topics

Chapter 28

# Leadership, teamwork and organizational dynamics

*William Elder Jr and Pablo Gonzalez Blasco*

Leadership is a common theme in many movies. The subject in such films is often the leadership style itself, with each style representing a stereotype. Patton comes to mind as an inspirational and autocratic leader. The Godfather was ruthless. Ghandi exemplified principled action and self-sacrifice. Audie Murphy 'led the charge.' This chapter uses scenes from several movies to provide examples of effective leadership, teamwork and organizational dynamics.

## Leadership under pressure

◆ *Apollo 13* (Tom Hanks, Gary Sinise, Kevin Bacon, Bill Paxton). With the words 'Houston, we've got a problem,' a moon mission ignored by most Americans as routine became a crisis in space. This true story exemplifies unconventional leadership styles in which leaders neither tell people what to do nor lead by example. Rather, the movie illustrates superb teamwork, both among the team in space and by the support personnel on the ground. Despite experiencing incredible physical and emotional stress, everyone involved in this flight demonstrates good communication skills and effective problem solving. Roles, responsibilities and leadership hierarchies are all well defined and executed with precision.

a (0:19:47–0:23:56). A sick team member is replaced with the consent of the team leader. 'This was my call.'

1 What are the responsibilities of a leader? How do these responsibilities differ from those of subordinates?
2 What effective leadership qualities are demonstrated by Tom Hanks' character?

b (0:50:10–1:00:03). Starting with an explosion in the tanks, things go seriously wrong on the *Apollo 13* spacecraft. In these scenes we witness physical, emotional and behavioral signs of stress. Project, mission and spacecraft commanders all demonstrate excellent communication skills, awareness of roles, responsibilities and individual strengths, as well as rational problem-solving techniques.

1 What signs of stress are evident among the crew members and the ground team?
2 Who are the leaders in these scenes? How do they handle their own stress and that of their subordinates? How is leadership demonstrated in these scenes? What are some qualities of good leaders?

3   What roles do the subordinates play? What responsibilities come with these roles? How well defined are everyone's responsibilities?
4   What aspects of these scenes illustrate good teamwork? How do effective leadership, clear role structure and accountability contribute to the outcome of the event? Are there any generalizations that you might draw from these scenes about healthy as opposed to unhealthy organizational dynamics?
5   How do the leaders help to solve the problem at hand? How do the subordinates help to solve the problem?
6   What movies have you seen previously that address leadership? What unique leadership styles are reflected in these movies?
7   Are there stereotypes for leaders? How accurate are these stereotypes? Have you encountered leadership styles that did not conform to the stereotype?

## Group process and leadership

◆ *Twelve Angry Men* (Henry Fonda, Jack Klugman, Lee J Cobb). This is an exemplary story about group process and the power of one person to change group outcome. Twelve jurors have to decide the guilt or innocence of a 17-year-old accused of killing his father. It is the hottest day of the year and the courtroom fan is not working. Eleven jurors vote guilty in an 'open-and-shut case.' Henry Fonda's character has the thankless role of the lone 'holdout.' He is not convinced by the argument of the other jurors, and raises questions that they do not wish to hear. Critical thinking, assertive communication and refusal to be intimidated are essential features of Fonda's character's leadership style. Most of the roles evident in group process are portrayed (bigot, clown, attention seeker, scapegoat, 'mouse' and emotional reactor).

a (0:04:00–0:14:16). This sequence of scenes shows the jurors socializing, organizing themselves to take the first vote and disagreeing when Fonda's character expresses concern that they may be too hasty in rushing to judgement.

1   Group roles often emerge during the early stages of group process. What roles do you see emerging among the jurors during this scene?
2   What leadership style do you see the foreman (played by a young Ernest Borgnine) demonstrate? What other leadership styles might the foreman have adopted? How do group members support the foreman?
3   Are all of the 11 jurors initially voting to convict equally sure of their position? What do you observe?
4   Distinguish between formal and informal leaders.
5   How does Fonda's character communicate his opinion in such a way as to avoid antagonizing other jurors?

b (0:38:00–0:39:00). In this scene Fonda's character takes a contrary position to the group, asks probing questions and disrupts a tic-tac-toe game.

1   What role does critical thinking play in Fonda's character's informal leadership style?
2   What personal characteristics are necessary for leaders to maintain an unpopular position despite strong social pressure to change that position? When does confident leadership cross the line and become arrogant leadership?

c (0:49:36–0:57:18). 'Eight to four.' A critical vote is taken in which some opinions have shifted among the jurors. Henry Fonda's character attempts to explain that certain facts in the case do not add up. This leads to an emotional confrontation between Fonda's character and that of Lee J Cobb.

1 What group process roles emerge in this scene?
2 What *intrapersonal* issues have to be resolved for the group to progress? What *interpersonal* issues have to be resolved for the group to progress?
3 What emotions emerge in this scene? What impact do these emotions have on the group process?
4 How well does the group manage conflict? How do groups best handle a 'rotten apple' in their midst? If you were the leader of this group, how would you proceed from this point onward?
5 Have you ever taken part in a group discussion? How did the group members attempt to influence each other?

## Leadership and self-sacrifice

◆ *The Patriot* (Mel Gibson). In this movie about the Revolutionary War, Benjamin (Mel Gibson) is an officer in the Colonial Army whose adult son is killed in action.

a (02:13:55–02:15:40). Grieving the loss of his son, Benjamin is ready to quit the war. His friend and fellow officer (Chris Cooper) asks him to stay and lead the upcoming battle. As Benjamin picks up and rides with his fallen son's flag, a crowd of beaten and wounded soldiers are inspired and become an army again.

b (02:26:17–02:28:00). In the midst of retreat, Benjamin throws away his gun, picks up the flag and with this action inspires his soldiers who, in turn, win the battle.

1 At what point do leaders 'belong' more to their subordinates than to themselves?
2 How are symbols, such as flags, used by leaders to motivate others?
3 Why are leaders' actions often more useful than their words in motivating subordinates?

◆ *Glory* (Matthew Broderick, Denzel Washington, Morgan Freeman). A movie about an African-American regiment (the 54th of Massachusetts) fighting for the North in the Civil War. Colonel Robert Shaw (Matthew Broderick) is their Caucasian commanding officer.

a (0:50:36–0:51:55). The regiment rebels against the Army's offer of 'slave' wages by refusing the money. Colonel Shaw observes their action and joins their refusal.

1 What does Colonel Shaw's behavior say about his ability to manage risk and self-sacrifice? Will his actions facilitate closer bonding with his regiment? Why or why not?
2 How important is it for leaders to be role models for their subordinates?

# Leadership and courage

◆ *Glory* (Matthew Broderick, Denzel Washington, Morgan Freeman). See previous section on leadership and self-sacrifice for movie description.

a (0:1:27:40–1:30:00). Colonel Shaw (Matthew Broderick) and a General discuss the strategic importance of quickly attacking Fort Wagner. However, only one regiment can attack at a time and it is likely that the first regiment to attack will suffer many losses. Despite their lack of sleep, Colonel Shaw asks that his 54th of Massachusetts be given the 'honor to lead the attack'. He tells the General that there is more than 'rest in fighting, sir . . . there is character and strength of heart'.

1 What traits help leaders inspire courage, character and strength of heart in their subordinates? Does the presence of courage and character say more about the group or its leader?
2 How do leaders build group solidarity among subordinates?
3 How can traits like courage, character and strength of heart be found in the work of doctoring?

# Chapter 29

# Technological considerations

*Heather A Kirkpatrick*

## Video-cassette recorder (VCR)

Today's medical educator has several choices to make regarding how to share cinema clips with their learners. One method, with which most educators are already familiar, is the use of videotapes. These generally require a television monitor, a VCR and a tape of the film itself. Most VCRs in use today have some form of counter. Since VCR counters are not exact, you may need to adjust the counter time to the portion of the film that you would like to show. This is because all VCR counters are not calibrated similarly, and there will probably be differences between the one used to time the clips described in this book and the one you are using to teach.

Videotapes have the advantage of being easily purchased or rented. Most residencies and medical schools have a television monitor and a VCR that is easily available on which to view film clips. In order to fast-forward to the video scene you wish to use, we recommend that you first use your remote control to press the *counter reset* button. Pressing this button twice will set the counter to zero. You need to set the counter to zero at the beginning of the movie, which we define as occurring as soon as the movie studio credits appear (usually right after the warnings from the FBI about unlicensed usage). You can then press *stop* on your remote control, press the *display* button (also on your remote) and fast-forward. The screen will remain blank except for the counter numbers. Press *stop* when you reach the desired counter number. To actually see the movie while you are rewinding or fast-forwarding (which may be necessary in order to find the *exact* scene, as time counters vary from one machine to another), press *play* and then either press fast-forward or rewind on your remote control. You will see the movie being shown at a fast speed, but you can stop when the right scene occurs.

## Digital video disc (DVD)

Recent technological innovations allow more flexibility for showing film clips. These innovations use digital technology, a new alternative that is available in the form of digital video discs (DVDs). DVDs are played on a DVD player, which today can cost less than $100. Many libraries carry films on DVD, and most current and past films are available on DVD.

DVDs are a technological cousin of CDs (compact discs), with which most people are familiar. Audio CDs contain audio sounds that are digitally stored, while DVDs contain both digital video and digital audio data. From the computer world, CD-ROMs allow individuals to store software or data files in a digital format for use with a personal computer. A CD-RW is a blank CD that allows individuals to record software, data, audio and video information from their personal computer. All of these types of disc (CD, DVD, CD-RW) are the same size and look similar, but they require different 'readers/players' to access the information that is stored on them.

DVDs require a DVD player. This is usually a stand-alone machine, similar to a VCR, that is attached to your television by a cable. Like VCRs, there are DVD *players* and DVD *recorders*. DVD recorders are extremely expensive and are regarded as a specialty item. DVD players allow you to read existing DVDs, but do not allow you to record information on them. A relatively new trend is for computers to have a DVD/CD/CD-ROM/CD-RW drive, which can read all types of disc and record data on CD-RWs. You can fast-forward and rewind films in exactly the same way as you would using a VCR, using buttons on either the DVD player or its remote control. Counter times on a DVD player should match up fairly closely with the VCR counter times. DVD counter times begin with the studio credits, and this is the method that has been used to establish times in this book.

## Advantages to the DVD format

The advantages of using this format include superior quality of picture/sound and ease of use. Because the storage of video and sound is digitized, it achieves a higher quality and sharpness that is not available on videotape versions. Another advantage concerns wear and tear. Videotapes tend to wear over time with use, and can eventually break. They are also susceptible to warping or damage from extreme heat, and the data can be destroyed by magnetic fields with which the videotape comes into contact. DVDs are not so susceptible to wear and tear, and are resistant to heat and magnetic fields. With proper care, the DVD, and the video and audio clips that it contains will last for ever. In addition, DVDs require much less physical storage space, as they are much smaller than videotapes.

Another advantage of DVDs is the fact that they can store much more information than videotapes. This allows many extra features to be included, such as film analysis by those involved in the making of the movie, and deleted scenes that were not shown in the final theatrical version. Such information may be helpful in your presentations.

Finally, ease of use contributes to the superiority of DVDs. Because the information is stored digitally, you may skip to any portion of a film that you desire without the counter inaccuracy problems that are found in VCRs. Position markers can 'bookmark' points in a film, or you may rapidly forward or back up while watching a clip. This can save minutes in a presentation when you are using two or more clips from the same movie. Using DVDs in this way means that you do not have to copy scenes on to another tape as you might do with videotapes.

Furthermore, many laptop computers now have the capability to read DVDs. If your audience is small, you may be able to use DVD films on a laptop alone, without a television. For larger groups you can hook either a laptop computer or a conventional DVD player to a television or LCD projector.

# Frequently asked questions about DVD technology

What is the difference between digital and traditional video storage systems?

This question can be rephrased as a comparison between analog storage and digital storage. Examples of analog storage include vinyl records, cassette tapes, clocks and videotapes. VCRs record and report data on videotapes in analog via magnetic fields. The analog storage system processes information in a continuous stream, similar to a clock with hands moving continuously. When recording either video or audio information in an analog manner, the information is degraded (i.e. specificity is lost) both during the recording process and each time the information is read or played. In a digital storage system, information is collected at specific points in time and recorded in binary format, using a series of 0's and 1's. Because the 'reader' only has to distinguish between a 0 and a 1, the resulting information that is stored has a higher quality.

Audio CDs collect and/or display information 44 000 times per second, allowing for very precise measurements, and the information does not degrade over time. For example, a data piece in which a sound is measured at '3401' will be recorded as '3401' in analog storage. However, errors may cause it to be read as '3400' or '3403', or as even more erroneous values. Analog readers have difficulty in distinguishing between '3401' and '3400,' although they would have no problems with distinguishing between '3401' and '54 387,' because the difference is greater. In digital storage, '3401' would be recorded in binary format and the 'reader' would only have to distinguish the 1's from the 0's – a job that digital readers, such as computers or DVD players, can do very accurately. Therefore '3401' is always read as '3401.' Because data are stored in binary format, they are compressed, allowing storage of more data on smaller physical items.

Where can I obtain more information about the technology of DVDs?

A great website is www.dvddemystified.com/dvdfaq.html

Are there different types or categories of DVD?

At this point the answer is no. All films are released in a standard format that can be played/read on a standard DVD player.

Where can I find DVDs to purchase or rent?

DVDs are available for purchase or rent in most retail stores that stock videotapes. They can also be ordered from multiple sites on the Internet.

How much do DVDs cost?

In general they cost between $15 and $25 to purchase, and between $3 and $5 to rent. Many public libraries have extensive DVD collections that are available for borrowing at limited or no cost.

Can I copy portions of a movie on to another disc for later viewing?

Although the necessary technology for this may exist, it is not currently available to the consumer, which hampers the practical applications of this format. This is one area where videotapes may have the advantage. With some rudimentary videotape equipment (e.g. two VCRs and cables to connect them), you can tape selected clips all onto one videotape for later viewing. It is likely that as technology becomes increasingly digital, the consumer will be able to edit clips for later viewing. However, we strongly recommend that educators check with local legal resources to determine the legality of copying videotapes.

## Future trends

Certainly the future points to most information being stored in a digital format. Trends in home cinema viewing include increasing data compression so that more data can be stored on fewer (or eventually smaller) discs. At present one can purchase portable DVD/monitor players that run off batteries to play DVDs. There are also small portable DVD players/recorders available that copy and display video images, but they are not yet sophisticated enough to play an entire film. As technology improves, this will probably become possible.

Finally, history tells us that it is likely that the video-cassette format will eventually be phased out by the film industry (in a similar manner to the way in which record albums gave way to cassette tapes and CDs). As VCRs and film video-cassettes become more obsolete, rental agencies may convert to using only DVDs, or movie studios may only release films in DVD format. If you find that the film you wish to use is only available on DVD, most hospital media/technology departments should have the necessary equipment to copy the film from a DVD to a VCR tape. Alternatively, as mentioned above, as the cost of a DVD player becomes more and more economical, it may be possible for medical education departments to purchase one for their own use.

# Part VIII

## The future of cinemeducation

Chapter 30

# The future of cinemeducation

*Matthew Alexander, Patricia Lenahan and Anna Pavlov*

Movies are here to stay. Despite numerous predictions that the advent of new technologies, such as television and the personal computer, would make the cinema outdated, movies are now as popular (if not more so) as ever, and have increasingly gained a worldwide audience.

Similarly, *cinemeducation* is here to stay. A burgeoning number of educators in an increasing array of disciplines are using popular movies to accentuate learning. These efforts are well documented in this book. However, as we look to the future, it is useful to define the challenges and opportunities for cinemeducation.

One of the greatest challenges for cinemeducators is simply keeping up with new movies – a daunting task if one is trying to identify potential scenes from contemporary movies for teaching purposes. In fact, the editors of this book have adopted the maxim *'So many movies, so little time'* to describe our difficulty in finding the time to review dozens of new movies for inclusion in this work. However, incorporating new movies into the cinemeducation curriculum is essential if our work is to remain vital. The editors of this book believe that the best way for this to happen is through professional collaboration. If *all* cinemeducators were to pool resources and share their favorite scenes from new movies (as well as unidentified scenes from older movies), then the individual workload involved in identifying scenes from these movies would be dramatically reduced.

However, for such collaboration to work, there needs to be a central gathering place for newly reviewed movie clips. There are currently several outstanding websites devoted to movies and teaching, most notably one based at New York University, which is cited in Appendix 4. However, there is no current website that identifies *specific scenes* for teaching purposes. Because of this vacuum, we encourage interested readers of this book to consider forming a *cinemeducation network*. Members of this network would share scenes from new movies applicable for cinemeducation. A website would then be set up to serve as a clearing house for 'new scenes' and to further facilitate collaboration between cinemeducators.

For such a cinemeducation network to be successful, it must include cinemeducators from the broadest possible array of disciplines including, but not limited to, family medicine, internal medicine, pediatrics, psychiatry, dentistry, family therapy, social work, clinical psychology, public education, law and pharmacology. Too often educators in one discipline are unaware of curricular innovation in other disciplines. We encourage readers of this book to reach out to interested colleagues from other healthcare and related disciplines and encourage them to become part of this network.

Another challenge for cinemeducation is to demonstrate scientifically that this approach is valid. In Chapter 27, Dr Alexander presents the results of a survey of graduates of a family practice residency program which uses cinema as a teaching tool. His finding that graduates enjoyed cinemeducation and believed that it enhanced their behavioral medicine training needs to be compared with results from other programs utilizing cinemeducation. To help to promote future graduate surveys, we have included Dr Alexander's questionnaire in Appendix 2. If his questionnaire was to be used without alteration in other programs, it would standardize the results. However, if necessary the instrument can be revised to fit other programs.

Other studies might use criteria other than self-report (e.g. written or oral tests, observation of the clinical interview) to assess whether cinemeducation is a more useful teaching tool than more standard didactic approaches. Another focus of research might be cinemeducators themselves, who could be studied to assess whether or not use of cinemeducation increases their job satisfaction. In fact a recent article suggested as much, positing that the use of film-based assignments helps to prevent instructor burnout.[1]

A third challenge for cinemeducators will be to keep up with the continuing evolution of the medium. Just as DVDs are replacing video cassettes, it is a certainty that new technologies will eventually replace DVDs. Cinemeducators will need to become facile with these emerging technologies, as the opportunities far outweigh the challenges. DVDs, for example, make it possible to go immediately to a scene rather than fast-forwarding to the scene as one has to do with videotape. Similar improvements will come with advancing technologies.

Finally, there is the human dimension. Although movies offer fun, entertaining and effective ways of augmenting teaching, they can also trigger troubling emotions in viewers. Unpleasant responses may include vicarious traumatization, emotional flooding, and indignation at the stereotypes and generalizations that find their way into cinematic portrayals of the human condition. These emotional reactions may even be *heightened* by the use of short clips as opposed to entire movies. Cinemeducators need to be continually alert to such possible negative responses, and to address them compassionately when they arise. However, if successfully addressed, these troubling emotions create opportunites for rich learning and deep connection between teacher and student.

In closing, let us say that although it may sometimes seem that all of the great movies have already been made, it is a certainty that there is a plethora of powerful, innovative and inspiring movies yet to come. For cinemeducators, this is a future well worth waiting for!

## Reference

1. Maynard P. Teaching family therapy theory: do something different. *Am J Fam Ther* 1996; **24**: 195–204.

# Appendices

# Suggested readings

## Child development

### Parenting

- Brazelton TB, Sparrow JD. *Calming Your Fussy Baby: the Brazelton way.* Cambridge, MA: Perseus Publishing, 2003.
- Brazelton TB, Sparrow JD. *Touchpoints: both volumes of the nation's most trusted guide to the first six years of life.* Cambridge, MA: Perseus Publishing, 2002.
- Blackman JA. Children who refuse food. *Contemp Pediatr* 1998; **15**: 198–216.
- Leung AK, Robson WL, Lim SH. Counseling parents about childhood discipline. *Am Fam Physician* 1992; **45**: 1185–9.
- Leung A, Fagan J. Temper tantrums. *Am Fam Pract* 1991; **44**: 559–63.
- Fremont WP. School refusal in children and adolescents. *Am Fam Physician* 2003; **68**: 1555–61.
- Goldenring JM, Cohen E. Getting into adolescent heads. *Contemp Pediatr* 1988; **5**: 75–90.
- Berman HS. Talking heads – interviewing adolescents. *HMO Pract* 1988; **1**: 1–11.

### Developmental issues

- Greenhill LL, Pliszka S, Dulcan MK *et al.* Practice parameters for the use of stimulant medications in the treatment of children, adolescents and adults. *J Am Acad Child Adolesc Psychiatry* 2002; **41**: 26–49S.
- Szymanski ML, Zolotor A. Attention-deficit/hyperactivity disorder: management. *Am Fam Physician* 2001; **64**: 1355–62.
- Chan E. The role of complementary and alternative medicine in attention-deficit/hyperactivity disorder. *J Dev Behav Pediatr* 2002; **23**: S37–45.
- www.chadd.org; CHADD – Children and Adults with Attention Deficit Hyperactivity Disorder. Website has list of local chapters.

### Divorce

- Tanner JL for the Committee on Psychosocial Aspects of Child and Family Health. Parental separation and divorce: can we provide an ounce of prevention? *Pediatrics* 2002; **110**: 1007–9.
- Cohen GJ for the Committee on Psychosocial Aspects of Child and Family Health. Helping children deal with divorce and separation. *Pediatrics* 2002; **110**: 1019–23.
- Whitham C. *Win the Whining War and Other Skirmishes: a family peace plan.* Glendale, CA: Perspective Publishing, 1991.
- Rothchild G. *Dear Mom and Dad: what kids of divorce really want to say to their parents.* New York: Pocket Books, 1999.

### Foster care

- Kools S, Kennedy C. Foster child health and development: implications for primary care. *Pediatr Nurs* 2003; **29**: 39–46.

## Death of a parent

- Rosen EJ. *Families Facing Death: a guide for healthcare professionals and volunteers.* San Francisco, CA: Jossey-Bass, 1998.

# Life cycle approach to sexuality

## Adolescent sexuality

- Bacon JL. Adolescent sexuality and teen pregnancy prevention. *J Pediatr Adolesc Gynecol* 1999; **12**: 185–93.

## Infertility

- Leiblum SR, Aviv A, Hamer R. Life after infertility treatment: long-term investigation of marital and sexual function. *Hum Reprod* 1998; **13**: 3569–74.

## Erectile dysfunction

- Weeks GR, Gambescia N. *Erectile Dysfunction: integrating couple therapy, sex therapy and medical treatment.* New York: WW Norton & Company, 2000.
- Eyles AE. Sexuality issues and common sexual dysfunction: evaluation and management. In: D Knespar, M Riba and T Schwenk (eds) *Primary Care Psychiatry.* Philadelphia, PA: WB Saunders Company, 1997.

## Anorgasmia

- Maurice WL. *Sexual Medicine in Primary Care.* St Louis, MO: Mosby, 1999.

## Sexuality and breast cancer

- Henson HK. Breast cancer and sexuality. *Sexual Disabil* 2002; **20**: 261–75.
- Murcia M, Stewart B. *Man to Man: when the woman you love has breast cancer.* New York: St Martin Press, 1990.
- Phillips NA. Female sexual dysfunction: evaluation and treatment. *Am Fam Physician* 2000; **62**: 127–36,141–2.
- Rabinowitz B. Psychosocial issues in breast cancer. *Obstet Gynecol Clin North Am* 2002; **29**: 233–47.
- Tan G, Waldman K, Bostick R. Psychosocial issues, sexuality and cancer. *Sexual Disab* 2002; **20**: 297–318.
- Weiss M, Weiss E. *Living Beyond Breast Cancer: a survivor's guide for when treatment ends and the rest of your life begins.* New York: Time Books, 1998.

## Sex and disability

- Lemon MA. Sexual counseling and spinal cord injury. *Sexual and Disabil* 1993; **11**: 73–97.
- Nusbaum MR, Hamilton CD. The proactive sexual health history. *Am Fam Physician* 2002; **66**: 1705–12.

- Nusbaum MR, Hamilton C, Lenahan P. Chronic illness and sexual functioning. *Am Fam Physician* 2003; **67**: 347–54.
- Gagliardi BA. The experience of sexuality for individuals living with multiple sclerosis. *J Clin Nurs* 2003; **12**: 571–8.
- Sipski ML. Sexual function in women with neurological disorders. *Phys Med Rehabil Clin North Am* 2001; **12**: 79–90.

## Menopause

- King DE, Hunter MH. Psychologic and spiritual aspects of menopause. *Clin Fam Pract* 2002; **4**: 205–19.
- Sherwin B. Menopausal myths and realities. In: D Stewart and NL Stotland (eds) *Psychological Aspects of Women's Health Care* (2e). Washington, DC: American Psychiatric Press, 2001.
- Stotland NL. Menopause: social expectations, women's realities. *Arch Women Ment Health* 2002; **5**: 5–8.

## Sexual desire later in life

- Meston CM. Aging and sexuality. *West J Med* 1997; **167**: 285–90.
- Andrews M. Calendar ladies: popular culture, sexuality and the middle-class, middle-aged domestic woman. *Sexualities* 2003; **6**: 385–403.

## Alternative sexual subcultures

- Celenza A. Sadomasochistic relating: what's sex got to do with it? *Psychoanal Q* 2000; **69**: 527–43.
- Lane RC. Anorexia, masochism, self-mutilation, and autoerotism: the spider mother. *Psychoanal Rev* 2002; **89**: 101–23.
- Lowenstein LF. Fetishes and their associated behavior. *Sexual Disabil* 2002; **20**: 135–47.

### Other interesting readings for alternative sexual subcultures

- Marc B, Chadly A, Durigon M. Fatal air embolism during female autoerotic practice. *Int J Legal Med* 1990; **104**: 59–60.
- Byard RW, Botterill P. Autoerotic asphyxial death, accident or suicide? *Am J Forensic Med Pathol* 1998; **19**: 377–80.
- Levitt EE, Moser C, Jamison K. The prevalence and attributes of females in sadomasochistic subculture: a second report. *Arch Sex Behav* 1994; **23**: 465–73.
- Moser C. S/M (sadomasochistic) interactions in semi-public settings. *J Homosex* 1998; **36**: 19–29.
- Moser C. Paraphilia: another confused sexological concept. In: PJ Kleinplatz (ed) *New Directions in Sex Therapy: innovations and alternatives*. Philadelphia, PA: Brunner-Routledge, 2001.
- Moser C. Treating sexual minority patients. *San Fran Med* 1998; **71**: 23–4.
- Moser C, Lee J, Christensen P. Nipple piercing: an exploratory–descriptive study. *J Psychol Hum Sexual* 1993; **6**: 51–61.

## Sexual addiction

- Schaumburg HW. *False Intimacy: understanding the struggle of sexual addiction*. Colorado Springs, CO: Navpress, 1997.

- Carnes PJ. *Out of the Shadows: understanding sexual addiction* (2e). Center City, MN: Hazeldon Information Education, 2001.
- Kasl CS. *Women, Sex and Addiction*. New York: Harper and Row Publishers, 1989.

### Additional resources

- www.saa-recovery.org; Sexual Addicts Anonymous.
- www.sa.org; Sexaholics Anonymous.
- Sexual Compulsives Anonymous. 800–977-HEAL.
- www.recovering-couples.org; Recovering Couples Anonymous.

# Geriatric medicine

## Retirement

- Atkinson DR, Kim AU, Ruelas SR, Lin AT. Ethnicity and attitudes towards facilitated reminiscence. *J Ment Health Counsel* 1999; **21**: 66–81.
- Butler RN, Lewis ML, Sunderland T. *Aging and Mental Health: positive psychosocial and biomedical approaches*. Boston, MA: Allyn and Bacon, 1998.
- Kulik L. The impact of men's and women's retirement on marital relations: a comparative analysis. *J Women Aging* 2001; **13**: 21–37.
- Lees E, Liss SE, Cohen IM, Kvale JN, Ostwald SK. Emotional impact of retirement on physicians. *Texas Med* 2001; **97**: 72–4.
- Mineau GP, Smith KR, Bean LL. Historical trends of survival among widows and widowers. *Soc Sci Med* 2002; **54**: 245–54.
- Peterson CC. The ticking of the social clock: adults' beliefs about the timing of transition events. *Int J Aging Hum Dev* 1996; **42**: 189–203.
- Utz RL, Carr D, Nesse R, Wortman CB. The effect of widowhood on older adults' social participation: an evaluation of activity, disengagement and continuity theories. *Gerontologist* 2002; **42**: 522–33.
- Vaillant GE, Mukamal K. Successful aging. *Am J Psychiatry* 2001; **158**: 839–47.
- www.nia.nih.gov/health/resource/rd2001.pdf; Resource for Older People.

## Hospital discharge and planning

- Gallo J, Fulmer T, Paveza G, Reichel W. *Handbook of Geriatric Assessment* (3e). Frederick, MD: Aspen Publications, 2000.
- Cole MG, McCusker J, Dendukuri N, Han L. Symptoms of delirium among elderly medical inpatients with or without dementia. *J Neuropsychiatry Clin Neurosci* 2002; **14**: 167–75.
- Beers MH. Explicit criteria for determining potentially inappropriate medication use by the elderly: an update. *Arch Intern Med* 1997; **157**: 1531–6.
- Morris V, Butler R. *How to Care for Aging Parents*. New York: Workman Publishing Company, 1996.

## Falls

- Gallo J, Fulmer T, Paveza G, Reichel W. *Handbook of Geriatric Assessment* (3e). MD: Aspen Publications, 2000.
- American Geriatrics Society. Guideline for the prevention of falls in older persons. *J Am Geriatr Soc* 2001; **49**: 664–72.

- Tromp AM, Pluijm SMF, Smit JH *et al*. Fall-risk screening test: a prospective study on predictors for falls in community-dwelling elderly. *J Clin Epidemiol* 2001; **54**: 837–44.
- Parra E, Stevens J. *US Fall Prevention Programs for Seniors*. Atlanta, GA: Centers for Disease Control and Prevention, National Center for Injury Prevention and Control, 2000; www.cdc.gov/ncipc/falls/fallprev.pdf

## Late stages and death

- Petersen RC, Stevens JC, Ganguli M *et al*. Practice parameter: early detection of dementia, mild cognitive impairment. An evidence-based review: report of the Quality Standards Subcommittee of the American Academy of Neurology. *Neurology* 2001; **56**: 1133–42.
- Bonder B, Wagner M, Davis FA. *Functional Performance in Older Adults* (2e). Philadelphia, PA: FA Davis Company, 2001.
- Mace NL, Rabins PV. *The 36-Hour Day: a family guide to caring for persons with Alzheimer disease, related dementing illnesses and memory loss in later life* (3e). New York: Warner Books, 2001.

# End of life

- Limerick M. Communicating with surrogate decision-makers in end-of-life situations: substitutive descriptive language for the healthcare provider. *Am. J Hospice Palliat Care* 2002; **19**: 376–80.
- Periyakoil V, Hallenbeck J. Identifying and managing preparatory grief and depression at the end of life. *Am Fam Physician* 2002; **65**: 883–90.
- Selwyn PA, Arnold R. From fate to tragedy: the changing meanings of life, death, and AIDS. *Ann Intern Med* 1998; **129**: 899–902.
- Singer PA, MacDonald N. Bioethics for clinicians: quality end-of-life care. *Can Med Assoc J* 1998; **159**: 159–62.
- Wenrich MD, Curtis JR, Ambrozy DA *et al*. Dying patients' need for emotional support and personalized care from physicians: perspectives of patients with terminal illness, families, and health care providers. *J Pain Symptom Manage* 2003; **25**: 236–46.
- Werth JL Jr, Gordon JR, Johnson RR Jr. Psychosocial issues near the end of life. *Aging Ment Health* 2002; **6**: 402–12.
- Fallowfield LJ, Lipkin M. Delivering sad or bad news. *Lancet* 1993; **341**: 476–8.

# Post-traumatic stress disorder

- Walker PF, Jaranson J. Travel medicine: refugee and immigrant health care. *Med Clin North Am* 1999; **83**: 1103–20.
- Gavagan T, Brodyaga L. Medical care for immigrants and refugees. *Am Fam Physician* 1998; **57**: 1061.
- McPhee SJ. Caring for a 70-year-old Vietnamese woman. *JAMA* 2002; **287**: 495–504.
- Mollica RF. Assessment of trauma in primary care. *JAMA* 2001; **285**: 1213.
- Moreno A, Piwowarczyk L, Grodin MA. Human rights violations and refugee health. *JAMA* 2001; **285**: 1215.
- Kramer EJ, Ivey SL, Ying Y-W (eds) *Immigrant Women's Health: problems and solutions*. San Francisco, CA: Jossey-Bass Publishers, 1999.
- Berman H. Children and war: current understandings and future directions. *Public Health Nursing* 2001; **18**: 243–52.
- Butler RO. *A Good Scent From a Strange Mountain: Stories*. New York: Penguin Books, 1992.

## PTSD secondary to a motor-vehicle accident

- Delahanty DL, Raimonde AJ, Spoonster E, Cullado M. Injury severity, prior trauma history, urinary cortisol levels, and acute PTSD in motor-vehicle accident victims. *J Anxiety Disord* 2003; **17**: 149–64.
- Kaltman S, Bonanno GA. Trauma and bereavement: examining the impact of sudden and violent deaths. *J Anxiety Disord* 2003; **17**: 131–47.
- Magruder KM, Albanese R, Frueh BC, Arana GW. Post-traumatic stress disorder detection and management in primary care. *J Clin Outcomes Manage* 2003; **10**: 559–68.
- Vermetten E, Bremner JD. Olfaction as a traumatic reminder in post-traumatic stress disorder: case reports and review. *J Clin Psychiatry* 2003; **63**: 202–7.

# Anxiety, depression and somatization

## Depression

- Valenstein M, Klinkman M. Minor depression. In: D Knespar, M Riba and T Schwenk (eds) *Primary Care Psychiatry*. Philadelphia, PA: WB Saunders Company, 1997.
- Greden J, Schwenk T. Major mood disorders. In: D Knespar, M Riba and T Schwenk (eds) *Primary Care Psychiatry*. Philadelphia, PA: WB Saunders Company, 1997.

## Phobias

- Bourne EJ. *The Anxiety and Phobia Work Book: a step by step program for curing yourself of extreme anxiety, panic attacks, and phobias*. New York: MJF Books, 1995.

## Anxiety disorders

- Nesse R, Eyler E. Anxiety disorders. In: D Knespar, M Riba and T Schwenk (eds) *Primary Care Psychiatry*. Philadelphia, PA: WB Saunders Company, 1997.
- Leaman TL. Anxiety disorders. *Primary Care Clin Office Pract* 1999; **26**: 197–210.

## Somatization disorders

- Fedes A. Somatization; www.columbia.edu/~am430/somatization.htm
- Righter EL, Sansone RA. Managing somatic preoccupation. *Am Fam Physician* 1999; **59**: 3113–20.
- Servan-Schreiber D, Tabas G, Kolb NR. Somatizing patients. Part II. Practical management. *Am Fam Physician* 2000; **61**: 1423–8.

# Chemical dependency

## Alcoholism

- Enoch MA, Goldman D. Problem drinking and alcoholism: diagnosis and treatment. *Am Fam Physician* 2002; **65**: 441–7.

## Teenage drug abuse

- Bergmann PE, Smith MB, Hoffmann NG. Adolescent treatment, implications for assessment, practice guidelines, and outcome management. *Pediatr Clin North Am* 1995; **42**: 453–72.
- Hanson WB, Rose LA. Recreational use of inhalant drugs by adolescents: a challenge for family physicians. *Fam Med* 1995; **27**: 383–7.
- McGarvey EL, Clavet GJ, Mason W, Waite D. Adolescent inhalant abuse: environments of use. *Am J Drug Alcohol Abuse* 1999; **25**: 731–41.
- Oetting ER, Edwards RW, Beauvais F. Social and psychological factors underlying inhalant abuse. *Natl Inst Drug Abuse Res Monogr* 1988; **85**: 172–203.

## Prescription drug abuse

- Longo LP, Parran T, Johnson B, Kinsey W. Addiction. Part II. Identification and management of the drug-seeking patient. *Am Fam Physician* 2000; **61**: 2401–9.

## Geriatric substance abuse

- Blow FC (ed.) *Substance Abuse Among Older Americans: treatment improvement protocol.* Washington, DC: Center for Substance Abuse Treatment, US Government Printing Office, 1998.
- Fleming MC (ed.) *A Guide to Substance Abuse Services for Primary Care Clinicians. Treatment Improvement Protocol.* Washington, DC: Center for Substance Abuse Treatment, US Government Printing Office, 1999.
- Oslin D, Katz ER, Edell WS *et al.* The effects of alcohol consumption on the treatment of depression among the elderly. *Am J Geriatr Psychiatry* 2000; **8**: 215–20.

# Family violence

## Child abuse

- Campbell JC, Lewandowski LA. Mental and physical health effects of intimate partner violence on women and children. *Psychiatr Clin North Am* 1997; **20**: 353–74.
- Felitti VJ, Anda RF, Nordenberg D *et al.* Relationship of childhood abuse and household dysfunction to many of the leading causes of death in adults: The Adverse Childhood Experiences (ACE) study. *Am J Prev Med* 1998; **14**: 245–58.
- Higgins DJ, McCabe MP. Maltreatment and family dysfunction in childhood and the subsequent adjustment of children and adults. *J Fam Violence* 2003; **18**: 107–20.

## Emotional and physical abuse

- Salzinger S, Feldman RS, Ng-Mak DS *et al.* Effects of partner violence and physical abuse on child behavior: a study of abused and comparison children. *J Fam Violence* 2002; **17**: 23–52.
- Walker EA, Gelfand A, Katon WJ *et al.* Adult health status of women with histories of childhood abuse and neglect. *Am J Med* 1999; **107**: 332–9.

## Impact of childhood sexual abuse and adult functioning

- Coid J, Petruckevitch A, Feder G *et al.* Relation between childhood sexual and physical abuse and risk of revictimization in women: a cross-sectional survey. *Lancet* 2001; **358**: 450–4.
- Dickinson LM, Degruy FV, Dickinson WP, Candib LM. Complex PTSD: evidence from the primary care setting. *Gen Hosp Psychiatry* 1998; **20**: 1–11.
- Laws A. Does a history of sexual abuse in childhood play a role in women's health problems? A review. *J Womens Health* 1993; **2**: 165–72.
- McCauley J, Kern DE, Kolodner K *et al.* Clinical characteristics of women with a history of childhood abuse: unhealed wounds. *JAMA* 1997; **277**: 1362–8.
- Mullen PE, Fleming J. Long-term effects of child sexual abuse. *Issues Child Abuse Prev* 1998; **9**: 1–9.
- Roth S, Newman E, Pecovitz D *et al.* Complex PTSD in victims exposed to sexual and physical abuse: results from the DSM-IV field trial for post-traumatic stress disorder. *J Trauma Stress* 1997; **10**: 539–55.
- Wyatt GE. Child sexual abuse and its effects on sexual functioning. *Annu Rev Sex Res* 1991; **2**: 249–66.

## Cycle of violence and physical abuse

- Fogarty CT, Burge S, McCord EC. Communicating with patients about intimate partner violence: screening and interviewing approaches. *Fam Med* 2002; **34**: 369–75.
- Sherin K, Sinacore J, Li X *et al.* HITS: a short domestic violence screening tool for use in a family practice setting. *Fam Med* 1998; **30**: 508–12.
- Weiss E. *Surviving Domestic Violence: voices of women who broke free.* Salt Lake City, UT: University of Utah, Agreka Books, 2000.
- Burge SK. Violence against women. *Prim Care* 1997; **23**: 67–81.
- Campbell JC. Health consequences of intimate partner violence. *Lancet* 2002; **359**: 1331–6.
- Campbell JC, Webster D, Koziol-McLain J *et al.* Risk factors for femicide in abusive relationships: results from a multi-site case control study. *Am J Public Health* 2003; **93**: 1089–97.
- Hamberger LK, Ambuel B. Spousal abuse in pregnancy. *Clin Fam Med* 2001; **3**: 1520–40.
- Hutchinson IW. Substance use and abused women's utilization of the police. *J Fam Violence* 2003; **18**: 93–106.
- Wolf ME, Ly U, Hobart MA, Kernic MA. Barriers to seeking police help for intimate partner violence. *J Fam Violence* 2003; **18**: 121–9.

## Delusional stalking

- Brewster MP. Power and control dynamics in prestalking and stalking situations. *J Fam Violence* 2003; **18**: 207–17.
- Burgess AW, Baker T, Greening D *et al.* Stalking behaviors within domestic violence. *J Fam Violence* 1997; **12**: 389–403.
- Burgess AW, Harner H, Baker T *et al.* Batterers stalking patterns. *J Fam Violence* 2001; **16**: 309–21.

# Companion animal abuse

- Ascione FR. Battered women's reports of their partner's and children's cruelty to animals. *J Emot Abuse* 1998; **1**: 119–33.
- Arkow P. The relationship between animal abuse and other forms of family violence. *Fam Violence Sex Assault Bull* 1996; **12**: 29–34.
- Jorgensen S, Maloney L. Animal abuse and the victims of domestic violence. In: FR Ascione, P Arkow (eds) *Child Abuse, Domestic Violence, and Animal Abuse.* Indianapolis, IN: Purdue Research Foundation, 1999.
- Munro H. Battered companion animals. *Ir Vet J* 1996; **49**: 712–13.
- Ritter WL. The cycle of violence often begins with violence toward animals. *Prosecutor* 1996: **30**: 31–3.
- Sable P. Pets, attachment and well-being across the life cycle. *Soc Work* 1995; **40**: 334–41.
- Spencer L. Overcoming domestic violence: Purdue's petsafe program propels people and pets to protection. *J Am Vet Med Assoc* 1996; **209**: 1054.

# Child witnesses to intimate partner abuse

- Boehm R, Golec J, Krahn R, Smyth D. *Lifelines: culture, spirituality, and family violence. Understanding the cultural and spiritual needs of women who have experienced abuse.* Alberta: University of Alberta Press, 1999.
- Prochaska JO, Velicer WF, Rossi JS. Stage of change and decision balance for 12 problem behaviors. *Health Psychol* 1994; **13**: 39–46.

# Impact of substance abuse on intimate partner violence and childhood exposure to trauma

- Anda RF, Whitfield CL, Felitti VJ *et al.* Adverse childhood experiences, alcoholic parents, and later risk of alcoholism and depression. *Psychiatr Serv* 2002; **53**: 1001–9.
- Leadley K, Clark CL, Caetano R. Couples' drinking patterns, intimate partner violence, and alcohol-related partnership problems. *J Subst Abuse* 2000; **11**: 253–63.

# Family violence and homicide

- Coker A, Smith P, Bethea L *et al.* Physical health consequences of physical and psychological intimate partner violence. *Arch Fam Med* 2000; **9**: 451–57.
- Gerbert B, Caspers N, Milliken N *et al.* Interventons that help victims of domestic violence. *J Fam Pract* 2000; **49**: 889–906.
- Rodriquez MA, Bauer HM, McLoughlin E, Grumbach K. Screening and intervention for intimate partner abuse: practices and attitudes of primary care physicians. *JAMA* 1999; **282**: 468–74.
- Stiles MM. Witnessing domestic violence: the effect on children. *Am Fam Physician* 2002; **66**: 2052–8.
- www.cdc.gov/ncipc/; CDC/National Center for Injury Prevention and Control.
- www.ojp.usdoj.gov/vawo/; US Department of Justice.
- National Domestic Violence Hotline. 800–799–7233.
- www.pvs.org; Physicians for a Violence-Free Society.

## Sexual assault

- Rosenfeld J, Ellwood A, Lenahan P. Rape and the consequences of sexual assault. In: *Handbook of Women's Health: an evidence-based approach.* Cambridge, UK: Cambridge University Press, 2001.
- Sebold A. *Lucky.* New York: Little, Brown and Company, 2002.

## Elder neglect and abuse

- Fisher JW. The hidden health menace of elder abuse. Physicians can help patients surmount intimate partner violence. *Postgrad Med* 2003; **113**: 21–30.
- Shugarman LR. Identifying older people at risk of abuse during routine screening practices. *J Am Geriatr Soc* 2003; **51**: 24–31.
- Swagerty D. Elder mistreatment identification and assessment. *Clin Fam Pract* 2003; **5**: 155–69.

# Chronic illness

## Pediatric chronic illness, child and parental issues

- McDaniel SH, Hepworth J, Doherty WJ. Childhood chronic illness. In: *Medical Family Therapy: a biopsychosocial approach to families with health problems.* New York: Basic Books, 1992.

## Truth telling

- Buckman R. *How to Break Bad News: a guide for health care professionals.* Baltimore, MD: The Johns Hopkins University Press, 1992.
- Mitchell JL. Cross-cultural issues in the disclosure of cancer. *Cancer Pract* 1998; **6**: 153–60.

# Schizophrenia and bipolar disorder

## Schizophrenia

- Olfson M, Weissman MM, Leon AC, Farber L, Sheehan DV. Psychotic disorders in primary care. *J Fam Pract* 1996; **43**: 481–8.
- Goldman LS, Wise TN, Brody DS. *Psychiatry for Primary Care Physicians* (2e). Chicago, IL: American Medical Association, 2003.

## Bipolar disorder

- Susman J, Manning JS, Keck PE *et al.* Foundational treatment for bipolar disorder. Supplement to *J Fam Pract* 2003; www.currentpsychiatry.com/supp_0303.asp
- Jamison KR. *An Unquiet Mind: a memoir of moods and madness.* New York: Alfred A Knopf, 1995.
- Copeland ME, McKay M. *The Depression Workbook: a guide for living with depression and manic depression.* Oakland, CA: New Harbinger Publications Inc, 1992.

- Papolos DF, Papolos J. *The Bipolar Child: the definitive and reassuring guide to childhood's most misunderstood disorder* (revised and expanded). New York: Broadway Books, 2002.

# Interviewing skills

## Active listening

- Egener B. Empathy. In: MD Feldman and JF Christensen (eds) *Behavioral Medicine in Primary Care.* Stanford, CT: Appleton and Lange, 1997.

## Nonverbal communication

- Platt FW, Gordon GH. *Field Guide to the Difficult Patient Interview.* Baltimore, MD: Lippincott Williams and Wilkins, 1999.

## Interruptions

- Beckman HB, Frankel RM. The effect of physician behavior on the collection of data. *Ann Intern Med* 1984; **101**: 692–6.
- Coulehan JL, Block MR. *The Medical Interview.* Philadelphia, PA: FA Davis Company, 2001.

# The professional and personal self

## Medical education

- Balint M. *The Doctor, his Patient and the Illness.* New York: International Universities Press, 1957.

## Physician–patient interactions

- Charon R. Narrative medicine: a model of empathy, reflection, profession and trust. *JAMA* 2001; **286**: 1897–902.

## The impaired physician/work addiction

- Robinson B. *Chained to the Desk: a guide book for workaholics, their partner and children and the clinicians that treat them.* New York: NYU Press, 1998.
- Sotile WM, Sotile MO. *The Resilient Physician: effective emotional management for doctors and their medical organizations.* Chicago, IL: American Medical Association Press, 2002.

## The medical marriage and family

- Bush J. Taking time out. *Fam Pract Manage* 2002; **9**: 78; www.aafp.org/fpm/20021000/78taki.html
- Vaccaro PJ. Six ways to make play a priority. *Fam Pract Manage* 1999; **6**: 68; www.aafp.org/fpm/990100fm/balancing.html

## Motivating healthy lifestyles

- Botelho RJ. Patients with alcohol problems in primary care: understanding patient resistance and motivating change. In: MR Stuart and JA Lieberman (eds) *Primary Care. Clinics in Office Practice*. Philadelphia, PA: WB Saunders, 1999.
- Botelho RJ, Novak S. Dealing with substance misuse, abuse and dependency. *Primary Care* 1993; **20**: 51–70.

## Family dynamics

### Family systems concepts

- McDaniel SH, Hepworth J, Doherty WJ. *Medical Family Therapy*. New York: Basic Books, 1992.
- McDaniel SH, Campbell T, Seaburn D. *Family-Oriented-Primary Care: a manual for medical providers*. New York: Springer-Verlag, 1990.

### Destructive interaction patterns

- Gottman J, Silver N. *The Seven Principles for Making Marriage Work*. New York: Three Rivers Press, 1999.

### Family breakdown

- Davis MW. *The Sex-Starved Marriage*. New York: Simon & Schuster, 2003.
- Miller TA. Diagnostic evaluation of erectile dysfunction. *Am Fam Physician* 2000; **61**: 95–104.

## Leadership, teamwork and organizational dynamics

### Leadership under pressure

- Langewiesche W. Columbia's last flight. *Atlantic Monthly* 2003; **292**: 58–87. This article provides an excellent insight into 'real-world' leadership and teamwork issues during the Columbia Space Shuttle catastrophe of 1 February 2003. This article from a popular journal would work well in conjunction with the clip from *Apollo 13*.
- Taylor RB. Leadership is a learned skill. *Fam Pract Manage* 2003; **10**: 43–8.

## Ethics and human values

### Understanding pain and suffering

- Kushner H. *When Bad Things Happen to Good People*. New York: Avon Books, 1997.

# Cultural diversity

## African American

- Dula A. The life and death of Miss Mildred: an elderly black woman. *Clin Geriatr Med* 1994; **10**: 419–30.
- Massad LS. Missed connections. Piece of my mind. *JAMA* 2000; **284**: 409–10.

## Asian American

- Lee E. *Working with Asian Americans: a guide for clinicians.* New York: The Guilford Press, 1997.
- Hong M. *Growing up Asian American.* New York: Avon Books, 1993.
- Culhane-Pera KA, Vawter De, Xiong P, Babbitt B, Solberg M (eds). *Healing by Heart: clinical and ethical case stories of Hmong families and western providers.* Nashville, TN: Vanderbilt University Press, 2003.

## Deaf American

- www.nad.org; National Association of the Deaf.
- Barnett S. Cross-cultural communication with patients who use American sign language. *Fam Med* 2002; **34**: 376–82.

## European American

- McIntosh P. White privilege: unpacking the invisible knapsack. *Peace Freedom* 1989; July/August: 10–12.
- Pergamet K, Maton H. *Religion and Prevention in Mental Health: research, vision and action.* Binghamton, NY: Haworth, 1993.
- Koenig H, McCullough M, Larson D. *Handbook of Religion and Health.* New York: Oxford University Press, 2001.

## Lesbian, gay, bisexual and transgendered Americans

- Harrison AE. Primary care of lesbian and gay patients: educating ourselves and our students. *Fam Med* 1996; **28**: 10–23.
- Rankow EJ. Primary medical care of the gay or lesbian patient. *N C Med J* 1997; **58**: 92–6.
- Berry C. Asian values, family values: film, video, and lesbian and gay identities. *J Homosex* 2001; **40**: 211–31.

## Latino American

- Pachter LM. Culture and clinical care: folk illness beliefs and behaviors and their complications for health care delivery. *JAMA* 1994; **271**: 690–94.
- Weller SC, Baer RD, Glazer M *et al.* Regional variation in Latino descriptions of susto. *Cult Med Psychiatry* 2002; **26**: 449–72.

## Native American

- Coulehan JL. Navajo Indian medicine: implications for healing. *J Fam Pract* 1980; **10**: 55–61.
- Jorgensen JG. Comment: recent twists and turns in American Indian health care. *Am J Public Health* 1996; **10**: 1362–4.
- Mahoney MC, Michalek AM. Health status of American Indians/Alaska natives: general patterns of mortality. *Fam Med* 1998; **30**: 190–5.

## End-of-life issues

- Irish DP, Lundquist KF, Nelsen VJ (eds). *Ethnic Variations in Dying, Death, and Grief: diversity in universality.* Washington, DC: Taylor and Francis, 1993.
- Rosen EJ. *Families Facing Death: a guide for healthcare professionals and volunteers.* San Francisco, CA: Jossey-Bass Publishers, 1998.

## Gay, lesbian, bisexual and transgendered issues

- Rankow EJ. Primary medical care of the gay or lesbian patient. *N C Med J* 1997; **58**: 92–6.
- Berry C. Asian values, family values: film, video, and lesbian and gay identities. *J Homosex* 2001; **40**: 211–31.

# Medical error

## Medical error: the price to be paid

- Gallagher T, Waterman A, Ebus A, Fraser V, Levinson W. Patients' and physicians' attitudes regarding the disclosure of medical error. *JAMA* 2003; **289**: 1001–7.
- Institute of Medicine, Committee on Quality of Health Care in America. *Crossing the Quality Chasm: a new health system for the twenty-first century.* Washington, DC: National Academy Press, 2001.

## Errors in judgement

- Brazeau C. Disclosing the truth about a medical error. *Am Fam Physician* 1999; **60**: 1013–14.
- Christensen JF, Levinson W, Dunn PM. The heart of darkness: the impact of perceived mistakes on physicians. *J Gen Intern Med* 1992; **7**: 424–31.

## Communicating about error

- Wu AW. Medical error: the second victim: the doctor who makes the mistake needs help too. *BMJ* 2000; **320**: 726–7.
- Levinson W, Dunn PM. Coping with fallibility. *JAMA* 1989; **261**: 2252.
- Goldberg RM, Kuhn G, Andrew LB, Thomas HA Jr. Coping with medical mistakes and errors in judgment. *Ann Emerg Med* 2002; **39**: 287–92.
- Rosner F, Berger JT, Kark P, Potash J, Bennett AJ. Disclosure and prevention of medical errors. *Arch Intern Med* 2000; **160**: 2089–92.

# Complementary and alternative medicine

## Home remedies

* Eisenberg DM. Advising patients who seek alternative medical therapies. *Ann Intern Med* 1997; **127**: 61–9.
* http://vm.cfsan.fda.gov/~dms/fdsupp.html; *An FDA Guide to Dietary Supplements.*
* http://nccam.nih.gov/; National Center for Complementary and Alternative Medicine (NCCAM).
* Jonas W, Levin J. *Essentials of Complementary and Alternative Medicine.* Baltimore, MD: Lippincott, Williams & Wilkins, 1999.

## Diets and dietary supplements

* Weiger WA, Smith M, Boon H *et al.* Advising patients who seek complementary and alternative medical therapies for cancer. *Ann Intern Med* 2002; **137**: 889–903.
* www.cfsan.fda.gov/~dms/ds-savvy.html; *Tips for the Savvy Supplement User: making informed decisions and evaluating information.*
* Rakel D. *Integrative Medicine.* Philadelphia, PA: WB Saunders, 2002.

## Health beliefs

* Najm WI, Reinsch S, Hoehler F, Tobis J. The use of complementary and alternative medicine among the ethnic elderly. *Alt Ther Health Med* 2003; **9**: 50–7.
* Adler SR. Relationships among older patients, CAM practitioners, and physicians: the advantages of qualitative inquiry. *Altern Ther Health Med* 2003; **9**: 104–10.
* Egede LE, Ye X, Zheng D, Silverstein MD. The prevalence and pattern of complementary and alternative medicine use in individuals with diabetes. *Diabetes Care* 2002; **25**.

## Spirituality

* O'Hara DP. Is there a role for prayer and spirituality in health care? *Med Clin North Am* 2002; **86**: 33–46.

## Mind–body dilemmas in healthcare

* Bornschein S, Hausteiner C, Zilker T, Forstl H. Psychiatric and somatic disorders and multiple chemical sensitivity (MCS) in 264 environmental patients. *Psychol Med* 2002; **32**: 1387–94.
* Caccappolo-van Vliet E, Kelly McNeil K, Natelson B *et al.* Anxiety, sensitivity, and depression in multiple chemical sensitivities and asthma. *J Occup Environ Med* 2002; **44**: 890–901.
* Caress SM, Steinemann AC, Waddick C. Symptomatology and etiology of multiple chemical sensitivities in the southeastern United States. *Arch Environ Health* 2002; **57**: 429–36.
* Chircop A, Keddy B. Women living with environmental illness. *Health Care Women Int* 2003; **24**: 371–83.
* Hall SW. Idiopathic environmental intolerances. *Minn Med* 2002; **85**: 33–6.
* Taylor JP, Krondl MM, Csima AC. Assessing adherence to a rotary diversified diet: a treatment for environmental illness. *J Am Diet Assoc* 1998; **98**: 1439–44.
* Terr AI. Environmental sensitivity. *Immunol Allergy Clin North Am* 2003; **23**: 311–28.

# Gay, lesbian, bisexual and transgender issues

## Coming out to the self

- Reynolds AL, Hanjorgiris WF. Coming out: lesbian, gay, and bisexual identity development. In: RM Perez, KA BeBord and KJ Bieschke (eds) *Handbook of Counseling and Psychotherapy with Lesbian, Gay, and Bisexual Clients.* Washington, DC: American Psychlogical Association, 2000.
- Stronski-Huwiler SM, Remafedi G. Adolescent homosexuality. *Adv Pediatr* 1998; **45**: 107–44.
- Harrison AE. Primary care of lesbian and gay patients: educating ourselves and our students. *Fam Med* 1996; **28**: 10–23.

## Coming out to each other

- Borhek M. *Coming Out to Parents.* Cleveland, OH: Pilgrim Press, 1993.
- Henderson MG. Disclosure of sexual orientation: comments from a parental perspective. *Am J Orthopsychiatry* 1998; **68**: 372–5.

## Coming out to the parent

- Borhek M. *Coming Out to Parents.* Cleveland, OH: Pilgrim Press, 1993.
- www.pflag.org; Parents, Families and Friends of Lesbians and Gays (PFLAG).

## Coming out to the spouse

- Grever C. *My Husband is Gay: a woman's survival guide.* Berkeley, CA: The Crossing Press, 2001.
- Buxton AP. *The Other Side of the Closet: the coming-out crisis for straight spouses and families.* New York: John Wiley & Sons, 1994.
- www.ssnetwk.org; Straight Spouse Network.
- Cole SW, Kemeny ME, Taylor SE, Visscher BR. Elevated physical health risk among men who conceal their homosexual identity. *Health Psychol* 1996; **15**: 243–51.
- Harrison AE. Primary care of lesbian and gay patients: educating ourselves and our students. *Fam Med* 1996; **28**: 10–23.

## Conversion therapy

- Reynolds AL, Hanjorgiris WF. Coming out: lesbian, gay and bisexual identity development. In: RM Perez, KA BeBord and KJ Bieschke (eds) *Handbook of Counseling and Psychotherapy with Lesbian, Gay, and Bisexual Clients.* Washington, DC: American Psychological Association, 2000.
- Harrison AE. Primary care of lesbian and gay patients: educating ourselves and our students. Who are lesbians and gay men? *Fam Med* 1996; **28**: 10–23.
- Shidlo M, Schroeder M. Changing sexual orientation: a consumers' report. *Prof Psychol: Res and Pract* 2002; **33**: 249–59.
- Shidlo M, Schroeder M, Drescher J. *Sexual Conversion Therapy: ethical, clinical and research perspectives.* Binghamton, NY: Haworth Medical Press, 2003.
- White M. *Stranger at the Gate: to be gay and Christian in America.* New York: Simon & Schuster, 1995.

## Concealing identity

- Borhek M. *Coming out to Parents*. Cleveland, OH: Pilgrim Press, 1993.
- Harrison AE. Primary care of lesbian and gay patients: educating ourselves and our students. *Fam Med* 1996; **28**: 10–23.
- www.pflag.org; Parents, Families and Friends of Lesbians and Gays (PFLAG).

## Gender variant behavior

- Outreach Program for Children with Gender-Variant Behaviors and Their Families; pgroup@cnmc.org.
- www.dcchildrens.com/gendervariance; *Free Parent Guide: if you are concerned about your child's gender behaviors.*
- Brown ML, Rounsley CA. *True Selves: understanding transsexualism – for families, friends, coworkers, and helping professionals.* San Francisco, CA: Jossey-Bass, 1996.
- Stronski-Huwiler SM, Remafedi G. Adolescent homosexuality. *Adv Pediatr* 1998; **45**: 107–44.

## Bisexuality

- Hutchins L. *Bi Any Other Name: bisexual people speak out.* Boston, MA: Alyson Publications, 1991.
- www.binetusa.org; BiNet is an umbrella organization for bisexuality; they collect and distribute educational material regarding bisexuality.

## Suicide

- Stronski-Huwiler SM, Remafedi G. Adolescent homosexuality. *Adv Pediatr* 1998; **45**: 107–44.

## Hate crime and victimization

- Savin Williams RC. Verbal and physical abuse as stressors in the lives of lesbian, gay male, and bisexual youths: associations with school problems, running away, substance abuse, prostitution, and suicide. *J Consult Clin Psychol* 1994; **62**: 261–9.
- DuRant RH, Krowchuk DP, Sinal SH. Victimization, use of violence, and drug use at school among male adolescents who engage in same-sex sexual behavior. *J Pediatrics* 1998; **133**: 113–18.
- Stronski-Huwiler SM, Remafedi G. Adolescent homosexuality. *Adv Pediatr* 1998; **45**: 107–44.

## Moving beyond shame

- Matthews CR, Lease SH. Focus on lesbian, gay, and bisexual families. In: RM Perez, KA BeBord and KJ Bieschke (eds) *Handbook of Counseling and Psychotherapy with Lesbian, Gay, and Bisexual Clients.* Washington, DC: American Psychological Association, 2000.
- American Psychological Association, Division 44. Guideline 1. Psychologists understand that homosexuality and bisexuality are not indicative of mental illness: guidelines for psychotherapy with lesbian, gay and bisexual clients. *Am Psychol* 2000; **55**: 1440–51.

- Borhek M. *Coming Out to Parents*. Cleveland, OH: Pilgrim Press, 1993.
- www.sunysb.edu/affirm; Psychologists affirming their gay, lesbian and bisexual family. AFFIRM encourages open support of GLBT relatives. Website posts bibliographies on issues often overlooked, such as couple relationships, domestic violence, adolescence, aging, family and parenting.

## Aging, grief and losses

- Baron A, Cramer DW. Potential counseling concerns of aging lesbian, gay, and bisexual clients. In: RM Perez, KA BeBord and KJ Bieschke (eds) *Handbook of Counseling and Psychotherapy with Lesbian, Gay, and Bisexual Clients*. Washington, DC: American Psychological Association, 2000.
- Harrison AE. Primary care of lesbian and gay patients: educating ourselves and our students. *Fam Med* 1996; **28**: 10–23.

## Same-sex families and children

- Matthews CR, Lease SH. Focus on lesbian, gay and bisexual families. In: RM Perez, KA Bebord and KJ Bieschke (eds) *Handbook of Counseling and Psychotherapy with Lesbian, Gay, and Bisexual Clients*. Washington, DC: American Psychological Association, 2000.
- Silverstein LB, Auerbach CF. Deconstructing the essential father. *Am Psychol* 1999; **54**: 397–407.
- Harrison AE. Primary care of lesbian and gay patients: educating ourselves and our students. *Fam Med* 1996; **28**: 10–23.

## HIV/AIDS

- Mayne TJ, Acree M, Chesney MA, Folkman S. HIV sexual risk behavior following bereavement in gay men. *Health Psychol* 1998; **17**: 403–11.
- Mays VM, Cochran SD, Zamudio A. HIV prevention research: are we meeting the needs of african american men who have sex with men? *J Black Psychol* 2004; **30**: 78-105.
- Mason HR, Marks G, Simoni JM, Ruiz MS, Richardson JL. Culturally sanctioned secrets? Latino men's nondisclosure of HIV infection to family, friends, and lovers. *Health Psychol* 1995; **14**: 6–12.
- National AIDS Hotline. 800–342-2437.
- www.thebody.com; An AIDS and HIV Information Resource.
- www.apla.org; AIDS Project Los Angeles.

## Transgender

- Brown ML, Rounsley CA. *True Selves: understanding transsexualism – for families, friends, coworkers, and helping professionals*. San Francisco, CA: Jossey-Bass, 1996.

# Eating disorders

## Childhood obesity

- Seim HC, Pi-Sunyer FX. *Management of Obesity*. American Family Physician Monograph 2. American Academy of Family Physicians, Kansas City, Missouri.

- Kimm S, Obarzanek E. Childhood obesity: a new pandemic of the new millennium. *Pediatrics* 2002; **110**: 1003–7.
- Stephens M. Children, physical activity and public health: another call to action. *Am Fam Physician* 2002; **65**: 1033–4.
- Schlosser E. *Fast Food Nation: the dark side of the all-American meal.* New York: Perennial Books, 2002.

# Disabilities

## Autism

- Kabot S, Masi W, Segal M. Advances in the diagnosis and treatment of autism spectrum disorders. *Prof Psychol Res Pract* 2003; **34**: 26–33.

## Neurological disorders

- Brown C. *My Left Foot.* London: Mandarin, 1989.
- www.comeunity.com/disability/cerebral_palsy/resources.html; ComeUnity: Children's Disabilities and Special Needs.

## Deafness

- Bat-Chava Y. Diversity of deaf identities. *Am Ann Deaf* 2000; **145**: 420–8.
- Lane H, Bahan B. Ethics of cochlear implantation in young children: a review and reply from a deaf-world perspective. *Otolaryngol: Head Neck Surg* 1998; **19**: 297–313.
- www.nad.org; National Association of the Deaf.
- Barnett S. Cross-cultural communication with patients who use American sign language. *Fam Med* 2002; **34**: 376–82.

# Graduate questionnaire

Please respond honestly to the following questions regarding your behavioral medicine experience during your Family Practice Residency at Carolinas Medical Center. Your responses will be confidential and will help us to assess the current curriculum.

*Gender:* Male   Female
*Age:*
*Years in practice:*

Please circle the number along the continuum that most correctly corresponds to your assessment using the following general key:

*1 represents strong disagreement; 5 represents a neutral response; 10 represents strong agreement.*

1  The behavioral medicine curriculum was an important part of my residency training.

    1    2    3    4    5    6    7    8    9    10

2  The behavioral medicine curriculum has directly impacted on my clinical practice.

    1    2    3    4    5    6    7    8    9    10

3  The behavioral medicine curriculum has directly impacted on my personal life.

    1    2    3    4    5    6    7    8    9    10

4  The use of film clips increased my enjoyment of the behavioral medicine curriculum.

    1    2    3    4    5    6    7    8    9    10

5  The use of film clips improved my retention of behavioral medicine concepts.

    1    2    3    4    5    6    7    8    9    10

6  I would recommend expansion of the use of film clips in behavioral medicine seminars.

    1    2    3    4    5    6    7    8    9    10

Please write in any additional comments you have about either the behavioral medicine curriculum or the use of film clips in behavioral medicine. Thank you in advance for your response.

_____
_____
_____
_____
_____
_____
_____
_____
_____
_____

Matthew Alexander, PhD

# How to build your video library

Once the decision has been made to utilize cinemeducation in working with medical students and residents, the next question is how to acquire a sufficient number of tapes to incorporate appropriate topics into a lecture series. Fortunately, there are many films that can be utilized for more than one topic. For example, the film *Down in the Delta* can be used to discuss autism, dementia, cultural issues and family relationships. Many of the films that are listed in Appendix 4 will be found in more than one section for this reason.

Now is a great time to build your library of videos for cinemeducation. The transition to DVDs is taking place, and videos are less expensive than ever before. Major video rental franchises such as Blockbuster will transition to an all-DVD format within the next year or two. Therefore inexpensive 'retired' rental videos will be available for purchase.

In the meantime there are a number of other ways to enhance your video library:

- Amazon.com. When you log on to Amazon.com, icons will be displayed that will direct you both to low-cost videos and to DVDs. For example, a new copy of the classic movie *Casablanca* has recently been available for $4.99.
- Barnes and Noble (bn.com). This bookstore giant also offers special sale-priced videos and DVDs.
- Wal-Mart, Target and other large chain stores often have videos available at a sale price. Drugstore chains such as Walgreens frequently advertise individual videos for $3.99 or three for $10.00. Needless to say, the selection may be quite limited and may not yield much, but it may still be worth a try.
- Best Buy, Circuit City and other stores that specialize in electronics also offer a variety of videotapes and DVDs at reasonable prices.
- Videos that are hard to obtain may be available from Amazon or other online companies through a variety of sellers who have used copies available for purchase.

# Appendix 4

# Selected movies and related websites and references

The movies in this index are grouped by subject. Readers who are looking for a specific topic may be routed to a more global subject heading that will expose them to a wide assortment of movies directly and indirectly related to their specific topic.

## Selected movies

**Abortion**
See Ethics and Human Values
. . .
**Abuse**
See Domestic Violence . . .
**Active Listening**
See Interviewing Skills . . .
**Addiction**
See Chemical Dependency . . .
**Dual**
See Lifestyle Modification . . .
**Nicotine**
See Lifestyle Modification . . .
**Work**
See Professional and Personal
Self . . .
**Sexual** – See Sexuality . . .
**AD/HD**
See Child and Adolescent
Development . . .
**Adjustment Disorder**
See Depression . . .
**Adoption**
See Foster Care . . .
*Immediate Family*
**Adult Development**
See Divorce/Separation/
Remarriage . . .
*About Schmidt* (parents of
young adults)
*Betsy's Wedding* (young adult
children)
*Father of the Bride* (children)
*Guess Who's Coming to Dinner*
(young adult children)
*Hannah and Her Sisters*
(marriage)
*He Said She Said* (marriage)
*Look Who's Talking*
(pregnancy and young
children)
*Look Who's Talking, Too*
(pregnancy and young
children)
*Love Actually* (single adults)
*Mr and Mrs Bridge* (marriage)

*Nine Months* (pregnancy)
*Notting Hill* (single adults)
*Scenes from a Marriage*
(marriage)
*Shadowlands* (marriage)
*She's the One* (marriage)
*Sleepless in Seattle*
(engagement, dating,
remarriage, blended
families)
*Steel Magnolias* (young adult
children)
*The Step Mom* (remarriage,
blended families)
*This Boy's Life* (remarriage,
blended families)
*Tortilla Soup* (remarriage,
blended families)
*Under the Tuscan Sun* (single
adults)
*Waiting to Exhale* (single
adults)
*When Harry Met Sally* (single
adults)
*You've Got Mail* (single adults)
**Aging**
See Geriatrics . . .
*Affliction*
*Age Old Friends*
*A Song for Mother*
*A Thousand Acres*
*Calendar Girls*
*Cocoon*
*Complaints of a Dutiful
Daughter*
*Da*
*Dad*
*Driving Miss Daisy*
*Eat Drink Man Woman*
*Folks*
*Grumpy Old Men*
*Hanging Up*
*Harold and Maude*
*Harry and Tonto*
*I Never Sang for My Father*
*Interiors*

*In the Bedroom*
*Iris*
*Kotch*
*Marvin's Room*
*Mr and Mrs Bridge*
*Nothing in Common*
*On Golden Pond*
*Shower*
*Smoke Signals*
*Son of the Bride*
*Tatie Danielle*
*The Divine Secrets of the Ya Ya
Sisterhood*
*The Gin Game*
*The Perfect Son*
*The Straight Story*
*The Whales of August*
*To Dance With The White Dog*
*Tribute*
*Trip to Bountiful*
*Troublesome Creek*
*Where's Papa?*
**Agoraphobia**
See Anxiety . . .
**AIDS**
See HIV/AIDS . . .
**Alcohol/Alcoholism**
See Chemical Dependency . . .
**ALS**
See Disabilities . . .
**Alternative Medicine**
See Complementary and
Alternative Medicine . . .
**Alternative Sexual
Subcultures**
*Alive and Kicking*
*All About My Mother*
*An Early Frost*
*Beautiful Thing* (coming out)
*Before Night Falls* (Cuban)
*Better Than Chocolate*
*Big Eden* (concealing identity)
*Boys Don't Cry* (transgender)
*Boys In The Band*
*Cruising*
*Eyes Wide Shut*

*Who's Afraid Of Virginia Woolf*

**Child and Adolescent Development**
*About a Boy* (self-esteem)
*Baby Boom* (baby needs)
*Beavis And Butthead*
*Dennis the Menace* (misbehavior, punishment, AD/HD)
*Digging to China*
*E.T. the Extra Terrestrial* (malingering)
*Finding Forrester*
*House Of Cards*
*Kramer vs Kramer* (divorce, developmental issues, parent involvement)
*Life As A House* (rebellion, death of a parent)
*Lil Rascals*
*Look Who's Talking*
*Look Who's Talking II*
*Lovely And Amazing*
*Marvin's Room* (death of a parent)
*Nine Months*
*Silent Fall*
*Stepmom*
*The Boy Who Could Fly*
*The Four Hundred Blows*
*The Good Mother*
*The Quiet Room*
*What's Eating Gilbert Grape?*
*White Oleander* (foster care)

**Chronic Fatigue**
See Chronic Illness . . .

**Chronic Illness**
See Disabilities . . .
*As Good as it Gets* (asthma, pediatric chronic illness)
*A Thousand Acres*
*Awakenings*
*Duet for One* (MS)
*Flawless* (stroke)
*Frankie Starlight* (dwarfism)
*Go Now* (MS)
*Good Will Hunting*
*Marvin's Room* (caregiving, truthtelling, leukemia)
*Regarding Henry*
*Safe* (impact of chronic illness)
*Soul Food* (diabetes)
*Steel Magnolias* (diabetes, impact of chronic illness)
*The Body Beautiful* (CA, RA)
*The Eighth Day* (Down's syndrome)
*The Gift* (chronic fatigue)
*Wildflower*

**Cocaine and Addiction**
See Chemical Dependency . . .

**Complementary and Alternative Medicine**
*Believers*

*Doc Hollywood* (home remedies)
*Eve's Bayou*
*Jacob's Ladder*
*Lorenzo's Oil* (childhood)
*Medicine Man* (home remedies)
*Mesmer*
*Safe* (dietary supplements)
*Soul Food* (health beliefs)
*Terms Of Endearment*
*The Cure* (childhood)
*The Green Mile*
*The Madness of King George* (porphyria)
*The Road To Wellville*
*The Sum Of It All* (stroke)

**Conversion Disorder**
See Somatoform Disorders . . .

**Cosmetic Surgery**
See Eating Disorders . . .

**Cultural Diversity**
**African/African-American**
*12 Bucks*
*4 Little Girls*
*Amistad*
*Angel Eyes*
*Antwone Fisher*
*A Raisin In The Sun*
*Barbershop*
*Beloved*
*Bethune: Making Of A Hero*
*Boyz N The Hood*
*Bringing Down The House*
*Brown Sugar*
*Cry Freedom*
*Domestic Disturbance*
*Do the Right Thing*
*Double Jeopardy*
*Down in the Delta*
*Guess Who's Coming to Dinner*
*Hoop Dreams*
*How Stella Got Her Groove Back*
*Imitation of Life*
*In the Bedroom*
*Jungle Fever*
*Laurel Avenue*
*Lumumba*
*Malcolm X*
*Mississippi Burning*
*Monster's Ball*
*Nowhere in Africa*
*Prince of Tides*
*Radio*
*Remember the Titans*
*Sarafina*
*Sleeping with the Enemy*
*Soul Food*
*Ten*
*The Air Up There*
*The Color Purple*
*The Fighting Temptations*
*The Gods must be Crazy*
*The Gods must be Crazy II*

*The Syringa Tree*
*Waiting to Exhale*
*What's Love Got to Do With It?*
*White Men Can't Jump*
*X*

**Amish**
*Witness*

**Asian American**
*A Green Dragon* (Vietnamese)
*Come See the Paradise* (Japanese)
*Eat Drink Man Woman* (Taiwanese)
*Heaven And Earth* (Vietnamese)
*Picture Bride* (Japanese)
*Salaam Bombay* (South Asian)
*Snow Falling on Cedars*
*Split Horns* (Hmong American)
*The Scent Of Green Papaya* (Vietnamese)
*The Vertical Ray Of The Sun* (Vietnamese)
*Three Seasons* (Vietnamese)
*Two Daughters* (South Asian)

**Chinese American**
*Crouching Tiger, Hidden Dragon*
*Double Happiness*
*Eat a Bowl of Tea*
*Farewell My Concubine*
*Flower Drum Song*
*Joy Luck Club*
*Ju Dou*
*Not One Less*
*Raise the Red Lantern*
*Shower*
*The Blue Kite*
*The Girl from Hunan*
*The Good Earth*
*The Road Home*
*The Story of Qui Ju*
*The Wedding Banquet*
*To Live*
*Yellow Earth*

**European American**
*Far and Away*
*Keeping the Faith*

**Greek/Greek American**
*Captain Corelli's Mandolin*
*Eleni*
*My Big Fat Greek Wedding*
*Zorba the Greek*

**Hispanic/Latino/Cuban**
*All About My Mother*
*Believers* (Cuban)
*Buena Vista Social Club* (Cuban)
*El Norte* (Mexican)
*Guantanamera* (Cuban)

Frances
Harold and Maude
It's a Wonderful Life
Network
'Night Mother
Ordinary People (major
    depression)
Pleasantville
Raintree County
Safe (mood disorder)
Saturday Night Fever
Sophie's Choice
The Astronaut's Wife
The Bell Jar
The Big Chill
The Bone Collector
The Crying Game
The Deer Hunter
The Evening Star
The Fisher King
The Hours
The Last Picture Show
Thelma And Louise
The Slender Thread
The Snake Pit
This Is My Father
Vincent And Theo
Virgin Suicides
Water Drops on Burning
    Rocks
What Dreams May Come
What's Eating Gilbert Grape?
    (dysthymia)
Who's Afraid of Virginia
    Woolf?
Who's Life Is It Anyway?
**Diabetes**
See Chronic Illness . . .
**Dietary Supplements**
See Complementary and
    Alternative Medicine . . .
**Dieting**
See Lifestyle Modification . . .
**Di fficult Patients**
Alfie (histrionic, narcissistic)
American Gigolo (histrionic,
    narcissistic)
Analyze This (entitled
    demander)
Annie Hall (schizoid
    personality)
As Good as it Gets (entitled
    demander)
A Streetcar Named Desire
    (histrionic personality)
Bullets Over Broadway
    (histrionic, narcissistic)
Carnal Knowledge (narcissistic
    personality)
Catch Me If You Can
    (narcissistic personality)
Citizen Kane (narcissistic
    personality)
Fatal Attraction (dependent
    clinger)

Jerry Maguire (narcissistic,
    histrionic)
Leaving Las Vegas (self-
    destructive deniers)
Never Talk to a Stranger
    (dissociative identity
    disorder)
Patton (histrionic, narcissistic)
Shampoo (histrionic,
    narcissistic)
Stardust Memories (histrionic,
    narcissistic)
The Caine Mutiny (paranoid
    personality)
The Odd Couple (manipulative
    help rejector)
The Talented Mr Ripley
    (antisocial personality)
Wall Street (histrionic,
    narcissistic)
What About Bob? (dependent
    clinger)
**Disabilities**
See Chronic Illness . . .
28 Days (self-injury)
Abres Los Ojos (Open Your Eyes)
Afraid of the Dark
After Darkness
A Patch of Blue (blindness)
At First Sight
Birdy
Born on the Fourth of July
Broken Cord (fetal alcohol
    syndrome)
Bubble Boy
Butterflies are Free
Charly (mental retardation)
Children of a Lesser God
    (deafness)
Coming Home
Dance me to my Song
Digging to China
Dominick and Eugine
Down in the Delta (autism)
Floating Away
Follow Your Heart
Forrest Gump
Four Weddings and a Funeral
Frankie Starlight (dwarfism)
Frida
How to Kill your Neighbor's Dog
I Am Sam
Inside Moves
Jean De Florette
Johnny Got His Gun
Love Affair
Mask
Maze (Tourette's disorder)
Molly (mental retardation)
Moonstruck
Mr Holland's Opus
My Left Foot (cerebral palsy)
Nell
Niagara, Niagara (Tourette's
    disorder)

Open Your Eyes
Passion Fish (paralysis)
Rain Man
Regarding Henry
Scent of a Woman
Seventh Veil
Simon Burch
Sound and Fury (deafness)
Table for Five
The Best Years of our Lives
The Bone Collector
The Elephant Man
The Man Without a Face
The Mighty (mental
    retardation)
The Miracle Worker
The Other Side of the Mountain
The Sixth Happiness (brittle
    bones)
The Theory of Flight (ALS)
The Tic Code (Tourette's
    disorder)
The Waterdance
The Whales Of August
What's Eating Gilbert Grape?
Wild Hearts can't be Broken
**Discharge Planning**
See Geriatrics . . .
**Dishonest Patients**
See Personality and
    Dissociative Disorders . . .
**Dissociative Disorders**
See Personality and
    Dissociative Disorders . . .
**Divorce/Separation/
    Remarriage**
See Child and Adolescent
    Development . . .
Damage
Divorce His, Divorce Hers
First Wives Club
Immediate Family
Interiors
Kramer vs Kramer
Mr Mom
Mrs Doubtfire
Parenthood
Parent Trap
Prince of Tides
Stepmom
Ten
The Four Seasons
The War of the Roses
**Domestic Violence**
12 Bucks
Abuse
American Beauty
Angel Eyes
Bastard out of Carolina
Bliss
Double Jeopardy
El Crimen Del Padre Amaro (The
    Crime of Father Amaro)
Enough
In the Bedroom

The Rookie
Varsity Blues
White Men Can't Jump
Winning
**Stalking**
Never Talk to a Stranger
One Hour Photo
**Stroke**
See Chronic Illness . . .
**Stuttering**
A Thin Line Between Love and
    Hate
Broadway Danny Rose
Do the Right Thing
Harlem Nights
My Cousin Vinny
One Flew Over the Cuckoo's Nest

Paulie
Primal Fear
Romy and Michelle's High
    School Reunion
Stalag 17
The Shawshank Redemption
The Sixth Sense
**Substance Abuse**
See Chemical Dependency
    and Lifestyle Modification
    . . .
**Suicide**
See Depression . . .
Torch Song Trilogy
**Teenage Drug Abuse**
See Chemical Dependency . . .

**Tourette's Disorder**
See Disabilities . . .
**Transcendence**
See Ethics and Human Values
    . . .
**Transgender**
See Alternative Sexual
    Subcultures . . .
**Truth-telling**
See Chronic Illness . . .
**Weight Loss**
See Lifestyle Modification . . .
**Widowhood**
About Schmidt
Love Actually
Shadowlands
Sleepless in Seattle

# Related websites

- http://faculty.dwc.edu/nicosia/moviesandmentalillnessfilmography.htm From Daniel Webster College, this website includes an extensive list of films and references dealing with mental health issues.
- www.us.imdb.com The international movie database includes over 80 000 films that are listed according to subject.
- www.psychmovies.com This website addresses how Hollywood has portrayed psychopathology in films.
- www.allmovie.com A good resource for finding movies. This site provides summaries of the films listed.
- www.geocities.com/sportsmovies/SPMD_Theme_Index.htm This is an extensive list of sports films divided into themes, including aggression, motivation, competition, confidence, leadership and more.
- http://psychclerk.bsd.uchicago.edu/movies.html This is an excellent website that includes lists of movies with psychological themes as well as articles written about films and therapy.
- http://endeavor.med.nyu.edu/lit-med-db/about.html
- www.imdp.com
- http://aging.ufl.edu/apadiv20/cinema.htm
- http://azstarnet.com/health/elder/020716bernard.shtml
- www.ifilm.com
- www.reel.com
- www.frii.com/~Parrot/Films.html Joy's media file on mental illness. This includes films, television and literature resources.
- www.amazon.com Search VHS or DVD and then click on Browse Genres for an assortment of movie topics.
- www.disabilityfilms.co.uk This is an excellent site that categorizes films related to disabilities into 'major' films, where the disability is a prominent aspect of the movie, and 'minor' films, where the disability plays a lesser role. This website also lists films according to the type of disability. Subject areas range from autism and amputees to stuttering and disfigurement.
- www.cinematherapy.com

# References

- Anderson D. Using feature films as tools for analysis in a psychology and law course. *Teach Psychol* 1992; **19**: 155–8.
- Barr T. Eating Kosher, staying closer: eight motion pictures that depict Jewish culture. *J Popular Film Television* 1996; **24**: 134–44.
- Bergstrom J. *Endless Night: cinema and psychoanalysis parallel histories.* Berkeley, CA: University of California Press, 1999.
- Connor DB. From Monty Python to total recall: a feature film activity for the cognitive psychology course. *Teachi Psychol* 1996; **23**: 33–5.
- Crutchfield S. Film studies and disability studies. *Disabil Stud Q* 1997; **17**: 284–7.
- Dans PE. *Doctors in the Movies: boil the water and just say ahh.* Bloomington, IN: Medi-ed Press, 2000.
- Doidge N. Diagnosing the English patient: schizoid fantasies of being skinless and of being buried alive. *J Am Psychoanal Assoc* 2001; **49**: 279–309.
- Fleming M, Manwell R. *Images of Madness: the portrayal of insanity in the feature film.* Rutherford, NJ: Fairleigh Dickenson University Press, 1985.
- Fritz GK, Poe RO. The role of a cinema seminar in psychiatric education. *Am J Psychiatry* 1979; **136**: 207–10.
- Gabbard GO. *Psychoanalysis and Film.* London: Karnac Books, 2002.
- Gabbard GO. *The Psychology of the Sopranos: love, death, desire, and betrayal in America's favorite gangster family.* New York: Basic Books, 2002.
- Gabbard GO. *Psychiatry and the Cinema.* Washington, DC: American Psychiatric Press, 1999.
- Gabbard GO, Gabbard K. The cinematic psychiatrist. *Psychiatr Times* 1999; **16**: 1–6.
- Gordon A. It's not such a wonderful life: the neurotic George Bailey. *Am J Psychoanal* 1994; **37**: 1031–49.
- Greenberg HR. A field guide to cinetherapy: on celluloid psychoanalysis and its practitioners. *Am J Psychoanal* 2000; **69**: 329–39.
- Hesley JW, Hesley JG. *Rent Two Films and Let's Talk in the Morning: using popular movies in psychotherapy.* New York: John Wiley & Sons, 1998.
- Hyler SE, Schanzer B. Using commercially available films to teach about borderline personality disorder. *Bull Menninger Clin* 1997; **61**: 458–68.
- Klobas LE. *Disability Drama in Television and Film.* Jefferson, NC: McFarland, 1988.
- Norden MF. *Cinema of Isolation: a history of physical disability in the movies.* Piscataway, NJ: Rutgers University Press, 1994.
- Peske N, West B. *Cinematherapy: the girl's guide to movies for every mood.* New York: Dell Publishing, 1999.
- Peske N, West B. *Advanced Cinematherapy: the girl's guide to finding happiness one movie at a time.* New York: Dell Publishing, 2002.
- Rabkin LY. *The Celluloid Couch: an annotated international filmography of mental health professionals in the movies and TV from the beginning to 1990.* Lanham, MD: Scarecrow Press, 1998.
- Safran SP. Disability portrayal in film: reflecting the past, directing the future. *Excep Child* 1998; **64**: 227–39.
- Safran SP. Movie images of disability and war. *Remed Special Educ* 2001; **22**: 223.
- Schill T, Harsch J, Ritter K. Countertransference in the movies: effects on beliefs about psychiatric treatment. *Psychol Rep* 1990; **67**: 399–402.
- Smith CJ. Finding a warm place for someone we know: the cultural appeal of recent mental patient and asylum films. *J Pop Film Television* 1999; **27**: 40–7.
- Solomon G. *Reel Therapy: how movies inspire you to overcome life's problems.* New York:

Lebhar Friedman Books, 2001.

- Solomon G. *The Motion Picture Prescription. Watch this movie and call me in the morning: 200 movies to help heal life's problems.* Fairfield, CT: Aslan Publishers, 1995.
- Teague R. *Reel Spirit: a guide to movies that inspire, explore, and empower.* Unity Village, MO: Unity House, 2000.
- Wahl O. *Media Madness: public images of mental illness.* Piscataway, NJ: Rutgers University Press, 1997.
- Walker J. *Couching Resistance: women, film, and psychoanalytic psychiatry.* Minneapolis, MN: University of Minnesota Press, 1993.
- Wedding D, Boyd M. *Movies and Mental Illness: using films to understand psychopathology.* Boston, MA: McGraw Hill College Division, 1998.
- Wilson C, Nairn R, Coverdale J, Panapa A. Mental illness depictions in prime-time drama: identifying the discursive resources. *Austr NZ J Psychiatry* 1999; **33**: 232–9.
- Wilson W. *The Psychopath in Film.* Lanham, MD: University Press of America, 1999.

# Editors' top ten picks

## Matthew Alexander's Top Ten Cinemeducation Films

1 *What's Eating Gilbert Grape?*
2 *The Doctor*
3 *What About Bob?*
4 *Ordinary People*
5 *Hannah and her Sisters*
6 *When a Man Loves a Woman*
7 *Annie Hall*
8 *Sleeping with the Enemy*
9 *Doc Hollywood*
10 *The Dead Poets' Society*

## Anna Pavlov's Top Ten Cinemeducation Films

1 *Wit*
2 *The Doctor*
3 *Kramer vs Kramer*
4 *Life as a House*
5 *What's Eating Gilbert Grape?*
6 *About a Boy*
7 *Baby Boom*
8 *Drunks*
9 *Mr Jones*
10 *Analyze This*

## Patricia Lenahan's Top Ten Cinemeducation Films

1 *Night and Fog*
2 *Down Came a Blackbird*
3 *The Theory of Flight*
4 *Kids*
5 *Drunks*
6 *Iris*
7 *Radio Flyer*
8 *Down in the Delta*
9 *Real Women Have Curves*
10 *Soul Food*

# Index